Sand to Sky

Books by Pamela Ellen Ferguson

The Palestine Problem   1973

The Pipedream   1974

The Olympic Mission   1976

Dominion   1977

The Sacrifice   1981

Decoration & Design for the 80's   1983

The Self Shiatsu Handbook   1995

Take Five   2000

Books by Debra Duncan Persinger PhD

Survey of Adolescent Knowledge,
  Attitudes and Behaviors Regarding
  Sexuality and AIDS   1995

Marriage and Family Student Guide   1996

Marriage and Family Instructor's Manual   1996

Lessons from the Inside   1997

Sand to Sky

✦

Conversations with Teachers
of Asian Medicine

Pamela Ellen Ferguson
and
Debra Duncan Persinger, Ph.D.

iUniverse, Inc.
New York Lincoln Shanghai

Sand to Sky
Conversations with Teachers of Asian Medicine

iUniverse books may be ordered through booksellers or by contacting:

iUniverse
2021 Pine Lake Road, Suite 100
Lincoln, NE 68512
www.iuniverse.com
1-800-Authors (1-800-288-4677)

Because of the dynamic nature of the Internet, any Web addresses or links contained in this book may have changed since publication and may no longer be valid.

ISBN: 978-0-595-44515-8 (pbk)
ISBN: 978-0-595-70822-2 (cloth)
ISBN: 978-0-595-88842-9 (ebk)

Printed in the United States of America

Front cover painting *Reflections—Variations on the Cosmic Mandala*
By Karen Greathouse, LAc (acrylic on wood, 24" x 24")

Calligraphy of *Wandering, Kindness and Wisdom* by Yuxia Qiu, LAc

Dedicated to the spirits of two extraordinary women who beamed different lights into the world of Asian Medicine and had the selfless ability to touch and change lives in endless ways.

Christina Herlihy, PhD: (1950–2004), former CEO of the National Certification Commission for Acupuncture and Oriental Medicine (NCCAOM), who will always be remembered for the love, generosity, integrity, kindness and inspired leadership that brought out the very best in everyone surrounding her.

Anne Gray, BS, RT (T), LAc, MSOM, Dipl OM (NCCAOM): (1950–2007), Acupuncturist, Teacher, former specialist in Radiation Oncology, who blasted away cobwebs of conventionalism to teach and practice her rigorous and heartfelt version of Integrative Medicine.

Contents

Acknowledgments. xiii

Debra's Preface xvii

Pam's Preface xix

A: TEACHERS—HERE, THERE, AND EVERYWHERE

CHAPTER 1 Pushing the Envelope—Developing Cross-Cultural
Sensitivity 3
by Maryanne Travaglione

CHAPTER 2 From Chengdu China to Texas USA. 10
by Jamie Wu

CHAPTER 3 Going Beyond "Chinglish" 16
by Zheng Zeng

CHAPTER 4 Teaching and Testing 19
by Debra Duncan Persinger

CHAPTER 5 Gained in Translation—Shiatsu and Trauma
Workshops from Belfast to Vienna 26
by Pamela Ellen Ferguson

CHAPTER 6 Shiatsu and Counseling in Zurich 35
by Madina Bokoum

CHAPTER 7 Teachers We've All Known—the Best and the
Rest. 42
by Debra Howard

CHAPTER 8 Back from Burnout in Britain 51
by Carola Beresford-Cooke

CHAPTER 9   Quotes on Burnout from Around the World 54

B: THE WORKPLACE

CHAPTER 10   Creating a Shiatsu School in Berlin 65
        by Edith Storch

CHAPTER 11   Creating a Shiatsu School in Hamburg 68
        by Wilfried Rappenecker

CHAPTER 12   Creating Schools of Acupuncture in the USA. 72
        by Stuart Watts

CHAPTER 13   From Shiatsu in Canada to Butterflies in Sri
        Lanka. 79
        by Nancy van der Poorten

CHAPTER 14   Outreach Clinics for Disaster Areas and City
        Hospitals 83
        by Kathleen Golden

C: LOOKING EAST—FACING WEST

CHAPTER 15   Weaving American and Asian Medicine
        Together 95
        by Anne Gray

CHAPTER 16   Theater and Therapists—Developing Interaction
        Skills 100
        by Megan Cole

CHAPTER 17   The Prisms of Clinical Counseling and
        Communication. 107
        by Lorena Monda

CHAPTER 18   Ethics, Borders and Boundaries 116
        by Cherie Sohnen-Moe

CHAPTER 19   Building an Acupuncture Practice From
        Storefronts to Web Sites. 125
        by Karen Nunley

D: ECLECTIC METHODOLOGY

CHAPTER 20   The Alchemy and Art of the Demonstration 133
by Lindy Ferrigno

CHAPTER 21   The Value of Dojo Training in Asian
Medicine 140
by Jeffrey Dann

CHAPTER 22   Exploring Pulse Diagnosis 146
by William Morris

CHAPTER 23   Five Element Wilderness Walks—Grizzlies and
Quicksand 155
by David Ford

CHAPTER 24   Is that a Cream Pie in Your Face? Songs and
Stories in Foundations of Chinese Medicine 160
by Barbra Esher

CHAPTER 25   New Meridian Discoveries and Directions. 165
by Tetsuro Saito

CHAPTER 26   Roots, Stems and Leaves—Chewing on Chinese
Herbs 170
by Lesley Hamilton

CHAPTER 27   Reflections on Pioneering Chinese Physicians
From 5000 BC to 1911 AD 180
by Jan Ste Germaine

CHAPTER 28   What Makes a Great Diagnostician? Quotes from
Around the World. 187

References. 197

Additional Reading List. 201

Glossary 205

Afterword 209

Acknowledgments

Sand to Sky could just as easily be called *Journeys in the Joy of Teaching.*

We are both passionate about education and the art of teaching, and share eclectic experiences of teaching globally. We also combine several years of very different experiences of Asian Medicine, exam development, and teacher training. Our many conversations during a transition period for us both during 2006 inspired us to interview a couple of dozen innovative teachers we knew in Asian and Integrative Medicine, as we wanted to showcase and honor work of this kind in a unique way.

We both enjoy books and movies by and about teachers who have made amazing breakthroughs utilizing unorthodox methods, like *Dead Poets' Society, Freedom Writers, Teacher Man,* and *Tuesdays with Morrie.* However, too little is known about similarly inventive and maverick teachers in Asian Medicine. So we invited an unusual array of voices of teachers we knew personally, to share their stories with us in a series of conference calls and e-mail interviews. We chose a lively, user friendly Question & Answer format to match their spontaneity, and to extract the essence of experiences some of them were too modest to document in any other form.

Our selection is not intended to be the definitive statement on the way Acupuncture, Chinese Herbs and Asian Bodywork Therapy (especially Shiatsu) should be taught. Quite the contrary. *Sand to Sky* is a forum, a talking point, and a prompt for future discussions, workshops, and books to help train the next generation of teachers. The stories will also swivel like a weather vane in the winds between west and east. We hope they help teachers from China, Japan and Korea transition into the very different classroom dynamics of North America and Europe, and help Western instructors experiment with new ways of transforming ancient forms of medicine for the practical demands of the 21st century. Experienced teachers of all backgrounds will not only enjoy the anecdotes of colleagues, but acquire fresh ideas and methodology. Our collection will be invaluable for Teaching Assistants.

We also threw open our windows to a wide range of friends in Asian and Western Medicine to share thoughts on topics of endless debate, like *What Makes a Good Diagnostician* and *How to Avoid Burnout*.

We hope *Sand to Sky* will inspire schools to give more thought to formal teacher training, something that is surprisingly lacking in this field. We have all experienced the best and worst of instructors, including cross-cultural and linguistic misunderstandings around differences in scope of practice and teaching methods involving Asia, the USA, Europe, and the British Commonwealth. Transforming Asian Medicine for the West is a challenge. We showcase some provocative and humorous experiences as a way of offering constructive guidelines for teachers to avoid some all too common mistakes.

We have used the politically correct term "Asian Medicine" to honor Asian Americans who have campaigned to eliminate the term "Oriental" because of its offensive colonial connotations. We only use the term "Oriental" when it lingers in the names of certain associations and schools. To honor differences in pronunciation we use *Qi ("chee")* in chapters on Chinese Medicine, and *Ki ("key")* in chapters on Japanese Medicine. We also honor the Chinese preference for the term *channels,* and the Japanese preference for *meridians.*

In other areas of *Sand to Sky* we also found it vital to reflect training in psychosocial topics, and in practitioner/patient and teacher/student interactive skills—areas that are too often neglected by schools. We found it equally vital to showcase the outreach internships and pioneering treatments practitioners and teachers have given in disaster zones, like post 9/11 New York City, and in clinics for AIDS and survivors of trauma.

While honoring the formal demands of curricular and clinical procedures to train future Asian Medical practitioners, we relish the stories of those teachers who have developed dazzlingly simple methods to help students understand dense theory in a snap. Some use theatrical props such as wigs and masks to teach different pathologies, or use funny rhymes to teach Chinese Herbs, or use helium balloons to teach Yin and Yang flows of meridian *Qi.*

The title *Sand to Sky* was Debra's spontaneous reaction when she first saw Karen Greathouse's beautiful painting *Reflections,* prompting us to choose it for the front cover. Karen is a Mexico City and Austin based Acupuncturist and Artist, and the painting was inspired by her love of the mandala. *Reflections* faces patients as they walk into her treatment room in Austin, a most appropriate opening for the stories you are about to enjoy. We appreciate Acupuncturist and Calligrapher Yuxia Qiu for the beautiful way she crafted the symbols for *Wandering*, *Wisdom* and *Kindness* to catch your eye as you journey through this book.

We would also like to honor the great support of literary agents Edy Selman (New York), David Grossman (London) and Ruth Weibel (Zurich), and special thanks for the splendid support from Phil Whitmarsh, and the team at iUniverse.com.

Finally, this work would not have been possible without the willingness and generosity of the following teachers who shared their insights and experiences, joys and challenges with us in a series of late night calls and an endless flow of emails. Our deepest appreciation goes to—in alphabetical order—Carola Beresford-Cooke (Britain), Madina Bokoum (Switzerland), Megan Cole (USA), Jeffrey Dann (USA), Barbra Esher (USA), Lindy Ferrigno (USA), David Ford (USA & New Zealand), Kathleen Golden (USA), Annie Gray (USA), Lesley Hamilton (USA), Debra Howard (USA), Lorena Monda (USA), William Morris (USA), Karen Nunley (USA), Wilfried Rappenecker (Germany), Tetsuro Saito (Canada & Japan), Cherie Sohnen-Moe (USA), Jan Ste Germaine (USA), Edith Storch (Germany), Maryanne Travaglione (USA & Italy), Nancy van der Poorten (Canada & Sri Lanka), Stuart Watts (USA & Britain), Qianzhi (Jamie) Wu (USA & China), Zheng Zeng (USA & China).

Pam and Debra

Debra's Preface

Sand to Sky is a gift both from and to the Asian Medicine community I loved to serve. It is an expression of my gratitude that closes out one chapter of my life while simultaneously providing a way for others to begin new and exciting chapters in their own lives. The book is about extraordinary people and healing and the interconnectedness of both.

When I left the National Certification Commission for Acupuncture and Oriental Medicine (NCCAOM) at the end of 2005 I was not given the opportunity to thank everyone in Asian Medicine who allowed me to grow and flourish for a decade in their midst. I particularly wish to thank those who worked closely with me, especially during my time as interim CEO, and as Executive Director of Testing and Certification Services when we created six national exams in three languages for four different professional board certifications in Asian Medicine. *Sand to Sky* presents the perfect way for me to make a final dynamic and positive impact on your world, to channel something back to the community, and to inspire the practitioners of tomorrow.

Prior to my connection with Asian Medicine I was a teacher at high school in New Zealand and at university in the USA, and I taught teachers how to teach. Just as teachers change lives, so too does Asian Medicine and when the two are combined, the alchemy is powerful. Catching a glimpse into the transforming of students into healers under the guidance of passionate and creative teachers is inspiring. My reverence for Asian Medicine and the remarkable people who practice it has deepened and getting to know the contributors to *Sand to Sky* through their work and work styles has been enriching. As a result my knowledge base has broadened and my excitement for the future of the Medicine continues to soar.

During the evolution of this book, there are special people whose friendship, unconditional love, and support I would like to mention because of what they taught me—not necessarily about Asian Medicine—but about what is most important in life. First, my four-year-old daughter Olivia, who, rather than be neglected while her mum worked, would "do Shiatsu" on my back while I lay on the floor proof reading chapters. She is my dream come true. The following friends expressed all the qualities and characteristics most people strive to attain, in honesty, truthfulness, selflessness, integrity, loyalty and courage to do the right thing in the face of adversity and hostility. They are my wacky, wise and wonderful friends—Christine Abbott PhD, Terri Beres, Michael Chung, Barbra Esher, Andrew Gamble, Summer Herlihy MD, Mina Larson, Anne McChrystal, Thomas Öst, Andrea Peng, Adam Smith, Neel Tenali and Maryanne Travaglione; and from New Zealand, Lesley Hamilton (unrelated to chapter contributor), Brian Harcourt and Romie Saunders. Last but not least I must acknowledge my gifted, generous and phenomenal friend and co-writer Pam Ferguson, for teaching and sharing so much with me, including feasts of chocolate and giggles at any time of night or day.

We are all teachers and we are all students. *Sand to Sky* honors and appreciates both.

Debra Duncan Persinger PhD
Overland Park, Kansas 2008

Pam's Preface

Sand to Sky realizes my dream of celebrating and connecting teachers of Asian Medicine and especially the wonderful teams with whom I have worked in many world capitals since the early 1980s after I linked my career in journalism to a new career in Asian Medicine. I appreciate my initial grounding in Shiatsu from my first teachers Pauline Sasaki, Esther Turnbull, and Ohashi in New York City in the late 1970s and early 1980s. In Canada, I loved teaching with Jean Lecomte, Lise Ste-Marie MD, Elisabeth Reichel MD, Raymond Ricard MD, Suzanne Ricard RN, Claudette LeBlanc, (Montreal); Tet Saito, Kaz Kamaya and Nancy van der Poorten (Toronto).

As I started my European teaching in Switzerland in 1984 I honor those who planned my early workshops, Rosemarie Soltermann, Erika Bringold, Bernadette and Sonja Winiker, Sonja Jaussi and Kristin Stalder. My current workshops at *Kientalerhof* are thanks to Mario Binetti. I honor Nicole Lorengo, Madina Bokoum and Martine Lorber who helped grow our *Flying Ki Shiatsu School* for experimental workshops in Zurich. Many friends across Germany involved me in the evolution of their schools and visions and always welcome my controversial workshops. Matthias Wieck was the first to invite me to Berlin in the mid 1980s and he later pioneered a school in former East Berlin. Elli Mann-Langhof, Wilfried Rappenecker and Heide Kuhl created a network of schools, and I continue to teach for *Shiatsu Schule Hamburg*. Edith Storch (*Shiatsu Zentrum Edith Storch*) pioneered a school for women in Berlin where we train dozens of practitioners. Bernhard Ruhla (Dresden) asked me to teach annually for him after the Berlin Wall fell. I have also been blessed with great translators—Beate Johl, Anne Zimmerman, Rita Wolters, Anne Fredericksen, Evie Berens, Ting Kohler, Stefanie Weidner, Nicole Lorengo and Karin Gsoellpointer. Recently I've welcomed teaching in Spain (Paloma Parras), in Northern Ireland, (John McKeever), in Holland (Kaima Nelson Bowne and Aliet Rogaar), and for the *European Shiatsu Institutes*—in Munich (Klaus Metzner), Heidelberg (Anna Christa and Bruno Endrich) and Vienna (Roberto Preinreich).

In the USA, I honor my colleagues at the *Academy of Oriental Medicine at Austin*, and thank AOMA Founder Stuart Watts who brought me to Austin to be Dean of Asian Bodywork Therapy from 1996–2004, to teach among many fine Acupuncturists. I also honor a great team on the national board of the American Organization for Bodywork Therapies of Asia.

I honor my dearest friend and co-writer Debra Duncan Persinger. Debra and I bring totally different skills to *Sand to Sky*. I started to work closely with her on the groundbreaking Asian Bodywork Therapy exam development committee during her outstanding years as the NCCAOM's Executive Director of Testing and Certification Services. Debra and I struck an instant chord because of our international backgrounds, our love of teaching, a shared BritWit (including a passion for lime marmalade) and a commitment to the evolution of an ancient form of Medicine to meet 21st century demands. I value the sharply objective eye she focused on each word in this work. Finally I applaud my closest soul sisters who helped me survive cancer so I could continue to teach and write, namely Bernadette Winiker, Nancy Casey, and Jocelyn Thompson (aka Sophie Keir) of the McDowall-Thompson Foundation. Onwards in *Qi!*

Pamela Ellen Ferguson
Austin, Texas 2008

A: TEACHERS—*HERE, THERE, AND EVERYWHERE*

And the day came when the risk to remain in the bud became more painful than the risk it took to blossom.
—Anais Nin (Author and Diarist, 1903–1977) (1)

I have been impressed with the urgency of doing. Knowing is not enough; we must apply. Being willing is not enough. We must do.
—Leonardo da Vinci (Artist, Engineer, Anatomist, 1452–1519) (2)

KINDNESS—calligraphy by Yuxia Qiu, LAc

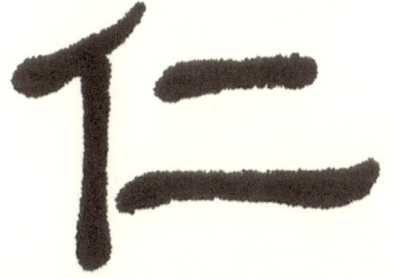

1

Pushing the Envelope—Developing Cross-Cultural Sensitivity

MARYANNE TRAVAGLIONE, LAc, Dipl OM (NCCAOM) *is a senior instructor at Touro College of Brooklyn New York, and a previous instructor at Mercy College and the Pacific College of Oriental Medicine, New York. She is also a former board member of the NCCAOM. Her first career was in theater. Maryanne is currently enrolled in a Doctoral program at the Oregon College of Oriental Medicine (OCOM) in Portland, Oregon.*

Q: Do your students have a rare opportunity to explore cross cultural diversity in your offsite clinics at Lutheran Medical Center of Brooklyn, New York?

MT: In one day at the hospital there are patients who speak Cantonese, Mandarin, Italian, Polish, Norwegian, Russian, and Spanish. The hospital has been mindful of cultural sensitivity around Chinese patients, like painting rooms pink and yellow instead of white, as white means death for the Chinese.

The multi-cultural staff reflects the neighborhood, and respectfully so. Our students work in Acupuncture services that are offered throughout in patient care at the hospital. We are most frequently consulted in neurology, Ob/Gyn, and oncology. We interact in many cultures and in many languages. We have access to translation services from the hospital, or family members provide the translation skill needed and in some instances for follow up cases. When necessary, our students use a Spanish dictionary to help them communicate with Hispanic patients. We are currently involved in a study where a medical anthropologist fol-

3

lows us around to see the ways in which alternative healers are being perceived in a hospital setting, how we interact with patients, doctors and nurses, and how students evaluate cases. She is collating her research for a future book.

We do our own paperwork for our school's clinical reports, and also report in the hospitals official records under consults with all the other medical departments. This is integration of care. We are treated as any other department consult in exactly the same way as any of the other official hospital services involving separate hospital notes.

Q: How have you been helpful in a cross-cultural challenge?

MT: My input helps with some of the Chinese patients, but I was also able to step in and help an Italian patient because I was the only one there that day that spoke Italian. She was refusing all physical therapy following knee replacement surgery until I discovered she was embarrassed because she hadn't showered for two days. She was also unhappy with the way the nurses were shaking her. Once we cleared up these problems, she was more than happy to accept physical therapy care.

My students and I always look at cultural taboos when discussing assumptions. For example, some cultures consider it inappropriate to talk about depression so you have to use careful questioning to find out if, for example, there may have been a recent death in the patient's family. On the other hand, if a patient claims to be depressed, I do not accept that as definitive, based on my definition of depressed. So I ask how it makes them feel and how they handle it. Similarly, I had a British patient who was perimenopausal and had a problem with the word "sweat." Later she described herself as "glowing in the dark," and she said, "only horses and laborers had sweat!"

Q: We hear you also had a very different sort of cultural exchange while trying to teach Qi to MDs at New York Medical College. What happened?

MT: I tried to explain the fundamentals of making *Qi*, but the MDs were having none of it. Finally a Chinese MD raised his hand and explained he would be able to describe how *Qi* was made as he understood both Western and Chinese Medicine. He talked about the absorption of food, and described *Jing Qi* in Chinese

Medicine as a type of catalytic activator where the inherited essence (Jing) stored in the Kidneys acted on the digestive system. He talked in a similar way to the way we talk about enzymes in Western Medicine. This is a very nice analogy that I have since used too. He then talked about the Spleen's role in making *Qi*. He did a very good job. But then one of the MDs challenged us by saying "we all know that the Spleen is not a digestive organ." The Chinese MD said, yes of course it's a digestive organ. But his colleagues were stuck on the idea that the Spleen was not a digestive organ and could not meet this culturally diverse explanation. The discussion ended here because the class had a certain prescribed set of knowledge to cover in a very limited space of time.

Q: On the flip side, Western students of Chinese Medicine feel that some of their Chinese instructors are too dismissive of symptoms like stress in patients.

MT: I don't find this to be a common problem but it takes a lot of cultural sensitivity. Some practitioners were taught to discount the spirit or the emotional body. We all have limitations and prejudices, and my advice is to turn this into a learning experience. Be respectful, ask questions, but learn something.

Q: How do you address all levels of cultural and ethnic customs and taboos among your eclectic mix of students?

MT: Well, how do you teach people to be culturally aware and sensitive? The answer is to keep talking about it. That's one of the wonderful things about teaching in New York, dealing with cross cultural diversity. Our students include Asians, Asian Americans, Hispanics, and East Europeans. We talk a lot about assumptions and I tell them if I say anything that insults anyone, please say so. I disclose my prejudices as they come up, but to do that I have to be aware of them. For example I treated a young Korean woman and made assumptions about her dietary changes, until she reminded me she had grown up on an army base in Korea and was raised on McDonalds! I bring this up when we discuss assumptions, and say how lucky we are in New York to be able to talk about issues like facial colors, race, privilege etc. I look around the room and see how many cultures are there and try to make everyone feel comfortable. But some people make assumptions about me, they assume "privilege" because I have a white skin. Until I remind them I grew up Italian in the South Bronx as a minority in my neighborhood.

Q: How do your students "walk the talk"?

MT: I encourage brown bag lunches to complete conversations that may arise in class and I also encourage a cultural and academic cross-mix of study groups, because this always encourages students to help one another. But we also discuss issues of power and balance and boundaries where this involves patients and teachers. Students commonly mistake dating patients as compassionate, but it isn't, because of the power differential. Similarly, it's equally inappropriate for students to date instructors.

Q: What procedures do you follow for teaching needling techniques for sensitive points?

MT: Firstly I set the stage. *Advanced Clinical Techniques* occurs at the end of the second clinical year. The students have already started treating patients in a clinical setting as assistants to senior practitioners. They have already practiced simple needle techniques and are building advanced clinical diagnostic assessment tools and clinical methods. In the *Advanced Clinical Techniques* class we go over clinical safety first. On the first day we not only go over OSHA safety and reinforce their clean needle technique which they learned in the basics class, but we move on to what I call the basic preparations necessary for a good practitioner.... Prepare self ... Prepare the environment ... Prepare the patient ... Prepare the Acupuncture point.... and then, finally one can Needle.

In preparation for the self we are able to discuss Self Development as a continued practice. We talk about personal development of our *Qi*, with any of the many types of *Qi* cultivation practices available for physical, mental and emotional growth and development in our personal and our professional lives.

Q: Once you've set the stage, what happens next?

MT: We tackle difficult techniques such as threading techniques, i.e., needles from GB 34 through to Sp 9, and then needle sensitive points such as Ht 1, UB 1 and Ren 1. We get to speak to our own fears of "hurting our patient" with strong sensations. We speak about ethical considerations around patient/practitioner boundaries and appropriate touch, and the inappropriateness of any personal patient/practitioner physical interactions. It becomes a perfect place to approach the topics of inappropriate sexual conduct, and what to do if feelings for patients arise. It is a valuable lab to bring to the surface why it is essential to maintain a professional relationship at all times with all patients. This allows the practitioner to use all the tools and Acupuncture points available in our medicine in effective ways.

In the end this class allows a young practitioner to learn the skills necessary not only to build skill around difficult points and sensitive areas of the body, but also to develop confidence around the basics of needling and draping techniques. They become comfortable in their interactions with difficult anatomical structures, working equally comfortably around arteries, bone, the eyes and the genital region. We teach only free-hand needling so this experience really develops skills that are losing ground in graduate schools in the USA. If we avoid teaching free hand needling because it is "less comfortable" for patients, we will lose, in my opinion, this very important part of our tradition. For this same reason, if we avoid teaching points such as Ren 1 and Ht 1 we lose this part of our tradition. You might as well take the points out of all our Acupuncture texts. This is a living medicine. We have a responsibility to keep these points and needle techniques alive and active and not allow them to be lost simply because we think they are unnecessary or difficult or embarrassing—or because they challenge our cultural taboos.

Q: So when you talk about creating a safe environment for this class, you mean both physical and emotional safety?

MT: It's as essential to create a safe, comfortable and respectful classroom as to create a safe, comfortable and respectful future clinical situation. So we talk about environments that are clean, safe and warm and allow a flow of *Qi*. For this reason the student can also understand more easily why inappropriate humor is not tolerated and why. Inappropriate joking with classmates or patients whom you are needling can be equally problematic. It really allows for a conversation about ethical considerations and interactions in very direct ways. As the students needle each other we have opportunities to discuss vulnerability and power dynamics in ways that I don't believe are possible when sitting in a purely didactic environment.

It is absolutely important that I teach appropriate draping and I also ask every practitioner I have ever met how he or she drapes Ren 1. I require students to be respectful. Any insensitivity in terms of behavior or inappropriate comments will not be tolerated. No student can opt out, every student has to needle and be needled on all the points. In one instance I had a class comprised of all males and one female. I made sure I stayed with the woman while she was being needled to make her feel comfortable. I advise students to get plenty of rest the night before, eat well, and dress appropriately, no sexually provocative underwear or anything like that. I also encourage students to palpate and needle themselves for practice. And I outline the specific reasons for needling Ren 1 (e.g., to stimulate urination after surgery).

Q: How were you taught to needle Ren 1?

MT: I was trained to needle it through underwear. But I teach Ren 1 as one of a series of *Sensitive Points* including Ren 22, St 1, UB 1, Du 1, Ht 1. And sometimes students are more concerned about UB 1 and Ht 1 than about Ren 1!

Q: Do you have a special way of teaching UB 1, GB 20 and Ht 1 to help students overcome fear and hesitation?

MT: I usually demonstrate and discuss the individual problems of each point and give one or two possible solutions. For instance with UB 1, I acknowledge how I approach what I say to the patient about why I want to use the point, acknowledge why it might be weird and ensure their comfort and consent. I always tell them to remind a patient of the possibility for bruising even if rare. In my opinion this is an important part of consent when needling on the face. I then demonstrate a technique for needling the individual point and then they pair up and I am all over the classroom with each individual, watching, supporting and encouraging their development of needling skills.

To watch and develop the confidence and skills of each student takes a lot of time but in my opinion brings the most reward. Many of the students have to develop their left hand, the palpatory and support hand. The classics refer to an Acupuncturist who knows how to develop the left hand as a superior practitioner, and in free-hand techniques this is essential. With each point in this class I get to observe a different aspect of needle technique and help the students explore ways for their development. From using a three inch free needle insertion at GB 30 to the steady hand needed for UB 1 and the slow strong advancing techniques necessary for a through and through—I always let them know that it takes many years of continued practice to perfect each point or technique successfully. In this class we can at least start engaging each student in the skills they can spend the next years exploring as they needle hundreds of points.

Q: What other sensitive issues have you encountered around needling?

MT: Some students go into needle shock. We then learn how to manage these clinical situations in a classroom, which hopefully will make them more comfortable in the future should this occur in a private clinical setting. And I had one student who could not bring herself to needle someone who had Quan Yin tattooed on her arms. The student could not needle the image of Quan Yin! So I moved her to work on somebody else. Another student had a problem with needling himself. He pulled my arm and said he used to be a drug addict, and hadn't used a needle on himself since quitting. I helped him work through the block by just offering to be there. Often that kind of support is all that is needed.

Q: What's one of the best examples of some dramatic aspect of your teaching that resonates with everyone, regardless of background?

MT: I tap out all the Pulses on a table, and engage the students by getting them to tap out Pulses, or tell me what they are reminded of when they feel those pulses or hear the sounds. I don't care if they don't know what this means.... they can just *feel* before they know what it all means. I teach Tongues and Pulses from Day One. We all look at a lot of tongues. I collect mirrors so they can look at their own tongues. I am very expressive and very interactive. And I enjoy moving around and staging the presentation. I have never taught a class sitting at a desk reciting from a scripted book. I usually have a desk filled with papers and articles and books and have a definite outline of what information needs to be included but will improvise the format depending on the dynamic of students involved.

2

From Chengdu China to Texas USA

QIANZHI (JAMIE) WU MD (China), LAc, AOBTA®-CI, *former Chief Acupuncturist, Chengdu University Hospital, China, former board member, NCCAOM, and currently Faculty Dean, and Director, Integral Studies, Academy of Oriental Medicine at Austin, Texas.*

Q: How long did it take you to adapt your teaching style from China to the USA?

JW: It took me about a year and a half to adapt!

Q: What sort of basic advice do you give your colleagues from China during their first week in the USA?

JW: Well, I share a lot of advice with them. Initially they need to polish their English. They might think they have good English until they arrive here and realize they don't understand students' questions. Instead of pretending they have understood, it's smart for them to ask students to repeat questions, and slow down.

Also, the school should have a training program and an orientation, and require the new instructors to sit in other instructors' classes. This is very important. The new instructors from abroad know almost nothing about teaching in the USA when they arrive, and should take orientation very seriously. They need to get a syllabus as soon as possible to familiarize themselves with the content. It took me about a whole year to prepare a teaching guide for all my courses. But then I felt more confident and found it easier to teach the same courses in subsequent years.

Q: How valuable have you found the "peer review" process involving all instructors, junior and senior, Chinese and Western, on an ongoing basis?

JW: The ongoing peer review system is vital. We sit in one another's classes and learn from other instructors. This strengthens communication. I learn many new teaching methods when I sit in other instructors' classes. This encourages all instructors to improve. After we review the feedback from others, we can recognize our mistakes. The peer review is just like a mirror. In short, the process helps mutual communication, evaluation and assessment.

Q: What other advice do you have for ongoing instructor training?

JW: We should continue to invite experts on higher education to give special workshops for faculty members, especially faculty from abroad, so that everyone is aware of the differences. And we should continue to invite instructors to give presentations and demonstrations in front of all faculty members. This is the best way of helping each other.

To help develop a multiple and comprehensive grading system, it's vital for instructors to revise their syllabi, to add new reading assignments for each class, and to create grading rubric systems for mind/body and Asian Bodywork Therapy courses. It's equally important to require students to write essays during most of the courses.

Q: How difficult is it to convince Acupuncturists from China—who are also Tuina experts—about differences in scope of practice in the USA where they may not use certain techniques (like neck and spinal adjustments) they were accustomed to using in Orthopedics in teaching hospitals in China?

JW: They need to know these and other legal issues as an Acupuncturist or Tuina practitioner. For example, they can't practice in their own clinic before they are licensed. They can't teach a practical course or supervise clinics until they get their temporary license. As a Tuina practitioner, they should never teach or demonstrate bone setting manipulations and spinal adjustments, even though they might have been practicing these daily in China.

Q: We hear that many instructors from China are initially shocked facing American students who ask questions, chew gum and prop their feet on the desk. How did you deal with this challenge?

JW: To tell you the truth, I was not used to it at the beginning. Chinese students respect their instructors very much because they learned the doctrine of Confucious and Mencius at middle and high school. American students don't have that background. Then I told myself that I should allow them more freedom in class. I even changed my own way of dressing to meet the new challenge. I don't wear ties anymore when I teach so that students feel more comfortable with me. On the other hand, I encourage students to ask questions, even when I taught in China. When students ask questions, you know where they are and what they need from you.

Q: Can you summarize the other major differences between students in China, and students in Master of Acupuncture programs in the USA who are of all ages and come from many different backgrounds and levels of education and other forms of training?

JW: Firstly, unlike American students, Chinese students do not need to work part time to support themselves and do not need to apply for student loans. They get supported by their families, who pay all their tuition, textbooks, apartments and pocket money. They just need to focus on their studies. A few students from the countryside may need to find minimal jobs. But most American students have to work to support themselves while they train. In short, Chinese students have more time to study.

Secondly, Chinese students are much younger and start their training at around 18 years. Most just graduated from high school and passed the required national examinations. They have endless energy and they memorize things quickly. Because they are all in the same age group, they are easier to teach. In the USA, the average age is much older, around 40, and ranging in age from early 20s to early 60s, which means instructors have to deal with a range of backgrounds and different learning skills. Older students tend to question more; they want to understand things before they can memorize them. In recent years, younger students are enrolling straight from college, but they're still older than Chinese students.

Thirdly, training in China takes longer than in the USA. A bachelor's degree takes five years, a master's degree takes three years, and a PhD takes another three years. That's a total of eleven years.

Fourthly, Chinese students have to memorize most classics, including *Neijing, Shang Han Lun, Golden Chamber* and *Warm Disease*. As I mentioned before, because they are young and they have good memories, they are accustomed to rote learning. Even if they don't fully understand the texts in that moment, they find them culturally easier to grasp in Chinese than an American can grasp them in translation.

And finally, Chinese students do not start their clinical practice until they have completed most of their courses in diagnostic and treatment procedures in Chinese and Western Medicine. Clinical internship happens in the last year. But American students often start their internship in the second year, even before they have finished Western pharmacology, Western diagnostic and physical assessment courses. Parallel training and clinic internship is arranged to make sure American students can get out of school in time and start to practice immediately to repay their student loans.

Q: Your students in America (who are from many different countries and backgrounds) praise and admire your teaching style because of the stories you integrate from your experiences as a Barefoot Doctor, your interesting assignments, your strong focus on Qigong and Tuina. Is this how you taught in China or have you expanded these methods for the USA?

JW: Storytelling from life and clinical experience always makes vivid and interesting teaching! Yes, because I was sent to the countryside for a year and a half towards the end of the Chinese Cultural Revolution and got the chance to collect raw herbs with a Barefoot Doctor, I'm able to share lots of stories. Students love to hear about the herbs monkeys chew in the mountains to rub on their scratches and injuries! As I have been practicing Chinese Medicine (including Herbs, Acupuncture, Tuina and Qigong) for over 20 years, I have many different stories to share about successful clinical experiences and observations. Students appreciate this as beginners as they need to *feel* this medicine, not just study this medicine.

When I was in China, I was not allowed to teach students Daoyin and Qigong at the beginning of my foundation classes, or even Tuina classes. But now I feel that stretching is so useful to help students focus and concentrate. They are always fresh, active, energetic and involved.

Q: What are your best methods for teaching Point Location and Point Energetics?

JW: The best method for teaching these courses is practice, practice and practice. The textbook suggests teaching the points channel by channel. But in my classes, I prefer to teach points region by region, not channel by channel. After I teach all the head points, I give students a whole three hours to review those points. I do the same for points on upper extremities, lower extremities, abdomen, back, and so on. In this way, students will not only learn the points for each channel, but also know point relationships on different channels. They will ask themselves questions such as—which acupoints on different channels are located at the same level of the umbilicus, or at the level of the second posterior sacral foramen, or are three cun above the wrist joint, and so on. In this way, students can really understand relationships among the points both horizontally and vertically.

Students often complain that it's hard to learn Point Energetics because many points have the same or similar functions, especially if they are on the same channel. I give them summaries of the general function of each channel, and then teach the differences among the points. Take Lung Channel as an example. All Lung Channel points release exterior syndromes, treat lung organ disorders, and treat Lung Channel disorders. Then Lu 10 and Lu 11 are especially good for an acute sore throat, Lu 6 is good for nasal bleeding and acute lung problems, Lu 9 helps tonify Lung *Qi* and so on. After students understand the common functions, only then can they understand the additional functions and differences. This can greatly help them understand and memorize Point Energetics, and especially help their clinical practice.

Q: How do you teach your students to activate Qi in a point before they needle it? Do you integrate some of your Qigong techniques first?

JW: Oh, yes. I teach students to feel *Qi* by applying Qigong methods. Point Location taught in textbooks and class is very general, very basic, but one dimensional. A real person could have a slightly different Point Location. The practitioner should be able to feel the differences by applying Qigong. The point is called *Shu* where *Qi* enters and exits. After we find the exact *Qi* point, we can definitely get better results. So *Qi* work is essential for locating acupoints, and achieving more effective clinical results.

3

Going Beyond "Chinglish"

ZHENG ZENG LAc, MD (China) *taught and practiced at Chengdu University Teaching Hospital China, and is currently Director of Acupuncture and a senior instructor at the Academy of Oriental Medicine at Austin. She also practiced and taught in Tel Aviv Israel. She specializes in gynecology, dermatology, and diabetes, has published widely on these topics, and on her clinical experiences and research treating psychoemotional problems.*

Q: How long did it take you to adjust to teaching in America?

ZZ: It took me about a year to adjust. Initially it was a big culture shock. Students kept asking the question *why* regarding topics related to Chinese Medicine. In China, students just try to memorize the information! But this is good for instructors, it makes us *think*. We also need to deal with cultural misunderstandings beyond "Chinglish." For example, in China, people understand the idiomatic use of language when we talk about someone having a "small gall bladder." It's not literal—it means they are very timid! But in America we need to explain this. I also need to explain to students that all points containing the word *Feng* (meaning "wind") expel wind, even when they are on different Channels. For example, Du 16 (*Feng Fu—Palace of Wind*) : GB 20 (*Feng Qi—Pond of Wind*) : GB 31 (*Feng Shi—Wind Market*) : UB 12 (*Feng Men—Wind Gate*).

Q: Many American students have problems learning Chinese Herbs (Single Herbs and Formulas). They find it hard to "memorize". Most like to smell, touch and taste the leaf, stem and root of Single Herbs, and to hear stories from their instructors about the clinical use of

Herbs. What have you found to be the best method for teaching Herbs to Western students?

ZZ: My teaching methods are different for first, second and third year students. During the first year I just teach them the pronunciation of Herbs. And to help them understand the different categories, I made a PowerPoint presentation to show them the plant, flowers, leaves, stem, and root. And I would give them key words to explain the different meanings. For example, the herb *He Shou Wu* (*Radix Polygoni Multiflori or Fleeceflower Root Polygonum)* contains the character *Wu* (meaning "dark/black"). The herb can prevent premature graying and help keep a patient's hair black (the root is dark brown/black). So the students could see the plant in color on the big screen and hear the words at the same time to help them make the connection. Actually *He* is a family name, so *He Shou Wu* means "Mr He's black hair!"

Q: What is the difference between the way you teach your Ob/Gyn classes in America, compared with the way you taught similar classes in China?

ZZ: There aren't big differences in the way we teach Ob/Gyn classes. We always treat according to symptoms and differentiation. I often teach through stories and case studies. For example, I share the story of an American patient who'd had two miscarriages and an abortion. She fell pregnant easily but we advised her to wait three months before trying to fall pregnant again after her last miscarriage. Her pulse was thin and weak in the Third Position. She had a pale purple tongue with a thick yellow coating. First we had to resolve Damp Heat, and to tonify and move Blood and resolve dampness. We also helped her rebuild Spleen *Qi* by advising her to avoid greasy foods and to eat more protein. We needled Sp 6, St 36, Ren 4, Du 4, Du 20. She took our advice, waited three months, fell pregnant and went to full term—with twins!

Q: Based on your own clinical experiences, what unique advice do you give students regarding needling and Herbs for common problems during pregnancy like morning sickness, insomnia, and depression?

ZZ: To treat—

- *morning sickness*—we encourage the patient to snap a rubber band against P6, and to sip peppermint tea or fresh ginger tea.

- *insomnia*—we encourage the patient to rub TaiYang and Du 20, and to place her feet in a bowl of warm water to calm herself and to bring the heat down from her head.

- *depression*—we use mainly Acupuncture, depending on the symptoms (usually *Qi* deficiency, Liver *Qi* stagnation, phlegm retention).

Q: And what points do you usually needle and teach for complications during pregnancy, like Hyperemesis (violent vomiting), tachycardia (rapid heartbeat)?

ZZ: To treat—

- *hyperemesis* (violent vomiting)—we needle St 36 and release a rubber band against P 6.

- *tachycardia* (rapid heartbeat)—we needle some points on the Heart or Pericardium channel and release a rubber band against P 6.

- But of course we also send them to their own Ob/Gyn. Mostly when there is violent vomiting, the patient has already visited their Ob/Gyn.

Q: What advice do you give your students about postpartum depression?

ZZ: Patients experiencing postpartum depression often need to be treated for Liver *Qi* stagnation or Spleen *Qi* Deficiency and Blood Deficiency because of the loss of blood and fluids during birth. So a good diet is important, and family support is also very important. In China there is often much more family support, enabling the new mother to have enough rest, which helps a lot. And women in China usually have only one child.

4

Teaching and Testing

DEBRA DUNCAN PERSINGER, PhD, DipTchg: *Executive Director, Federation of State Massage Therapy Boards (FSMTB), former interim CEO and Executive Director of Testing and Certification Services, National Certification Commission for Acupuncture and Oriental Medicine (NCCAOM).*

Q: *What was your first experience of teaching?*

DDP: At age three or four I got into trouble for using chalk on our closet doors as a blackboard to teach my imaginary students! In school I used to try and finish my work as fast as I could so I could help other kids in the class. At the age of 12, I loved visiting a special school once a week to work with intellectually challenged students aged between five and 16. My teachers all knew I was destined for a career in teaching.

Q: *Given your extensive training as a teacher, and your experience of teaching at high school in New Zealand and at university in the USA, what advice do you have for Teachers-in-training, regardless of subject?*

DDP: That one has to teach the people first and the subject second. To trust in themselves and their own abilities and not try to replicate the style of someone else. For example, during my Teacher training I had an inner struggle with a teaching supervisor over her insistence on demonstrating a nutritional breakfast of spaghetti and egg for Polynesian schoolchildren—something I considered a complete cultural mismatch with the students. Nevertheless, I stood back and let her be the Teacher with the supposedly model practices. I drew up a lesson plan that included her breakfast dish and submitted my assignment to the head of the department. I should have trusted my own instincts—the lesson was declared culturally inappropriate and I was encouraged to focus on improving cultural awareness. Teachers-in-training must be encouraged to be their own person, develop their own style, especially in situations where they recognize cross-cultural mistakes or assumptions. On the other hand, supervisors need to "read" teachers-in-training, communicate with them, be discerning, and not make quick assumptions based on perceived behavior. One supervisor labeled me as "apathetic" when I chose not to complete a specific project she had suggested. She didn't ask the next question to find out that I was dealing with two major family crises at the time that were a far higher priority than designing a display for the back of her classroom wall.

Q: *Where did the responsibility lie in both those instances? The supervisors for being insensitive? Or you, for being too polite, and too reluctant to speak up?*

DDP: I certainly take responsibility for not politely challenging the supervisor, if not for my own sake, then for the poor students who had to consume that horrible spaghetti and egg mixture! Incidentally, it was the same supervisor at the center of both of these examples. She taught me valuable lessons about what I did *not* want to be like as a teacher. Her responsibility lay in the fact that she did not respond to the needs of her students, nor did she do her homework to ensure that what she was teaching was accurate and relevant to the students' educational needs.

Q: *I heard you utilized a very unusual way of communicating with an aggressive student. Can you describe the incident?*

DDP: I noticed a teenager displaying physical and verbal aggression toward other students. Normally the classic way of dealing with him would be to punish him through detention. But I picked up a huge copy of the yellow pages telephone book, took him outside the classroom, and invited him to punch the book, hard. Which he did, several times. Then he started to cry and told me about the pain he was experiencing because his parents were going through a divorce. Although this case involved an adolescent and not the typical Asian Medicine student who might range in age from early twenties to early sixties, issues surrounding anger and other emotional manifestations do surface and teachers are not always equipped to handle the situations with sensitivity and care. This is why I am an advocate of quality teacher training and why such issues are highlighted in *Sand to Sky*.

Q: *During your interactions over the past decade with a wide range of instructors, practitioners and committees of Acupuncture, Chinese Herbology, Asian Bodywork Therapy, and Biomedicine, what other gaps in Asian Medical training did you notice during your discussions around the USA?*

DDP: A lack of uniformity, with variations in the way subjects are taught, and in methods of assessment. For example, many instructors do not know how to write a good test, which is understandable considering they are not trained to teach. By comparison, in New Zealand, I received my undergraduate degree in my subject matter and then spent a year of post graduate teacher training at a College of Education to receive my Diploma in Teaching. Ideally, I think formal teacher training would serve the educational institutions and individual academicians, and the students would obviously, and most importantly, reap the benefits as well. Also I noticed limited, if any, psychosocial training, and inadequate training in issues like transference, which is why we have addressed these topics in *Sand to Sky.*

Trainee psychotherapists are required to undergo personal therapy to help them address certain issues. It may be worthwhile for students of Asian Medicine to have similar requirements, especially to work through their own unresolved issues. Learning from other professionals, not necessarily limited to Asian Medicine, is invaluable. Much of the delicate nature of working with patients' emotions cannot be learned in a formal classroom setting, either because it is too structured, or the timing may not be right for some people to grasp the teachable moment. Much of this has to do with how a practitioner responds to crises in his or her life. It's equally important to teach potential practitioners exercises in self-protection. The helping professions are understandably prone to burnout and compassion fatigue, another vital topic highlighted in *Sand to Sky.* Asian Medicine practitioners who are also teachers need to be mindful of "walking their talk" in order to sustain the ability to treat and teach without being drained and overloaded.

Q: *What are some of the Ethical challenges that hit Asian practitioners in the West, especially in the USA?*

DDP: Most cross-cultural challenges arise from language barriers and being unfamiliar with certain practices including the detailed documentation required by insurance companies, issues of privacy and patient confidentiality, and issues of modesty like proper draping techniques. There are specific cultural considerations. For example, in some Asian countries the families are informed first about a patient's condition but this would be unlawful in the USA, without the patient's voluntary and signed consent.

To avoid potential conflicts, schools and group practices would be wise to offer detailed briefing sessions and informational lists of proper procedures, as required by national laws or state laws.

Q: Given your own background in a British style of education involving essays, and exam questions requiring analytical thought, not just factual knowledge, what is your impression of multiple-choice questions in the USA?

DDP: For the purposes of licensure and certification, multiple-choice items are invaluable for assessing the knowledge base for large populations of candidates. And certainly, due to the amount of fraud, I believe it is better to have a national assessment method rather than the limitation of just having to prove education and training. Multiple-choice assessment offers an efficient way of testing a wide range of issues succinctly, and can be reliably scored since all answers are predetermined. Computer scoring provides easy access to item analysis to pinpoint any potentially problematic items. Students are reassured that grading is far less subjective, although there is a certain amount of subjectivity in the choice of questions and options. There is also a distinct advantage for candidates for whom English is a second language because the assessment is not affected by the students' ability to write. Multiple-choice items can also reach a greater cognitive level than simple recall of facts. Many incorrectly assume that "the test" is the only component that determines licensure or certification when, in fact, the award of a license or certification is also comprised of meeting additional requirements such as the completion of a formal didactic and clinical education. So, a national examination is only one piece in the overall assessment of professional competence.

Q: *You've addressed the advantages of the multiple-choice format. But what are the disadvantages?*

DDP: Teachers are concerned that students may choose the right answer for the wrong reason, or make a lucky guess. If students are asked to explain their answers or weigh the evidence and defend a position or mode of treatment, as in a short answer or essay format, the teacher can spot the difference between a lucky guess and real knowledge. Multiple choice questions do not test the students' ability to develop and organize their ideas, or present them in a coherent argument. When the questions relate to treatments, the restrictions of only four or five options do not allow students to explore other clinical possibilities.

Q: *You've stated that most instructors have had little preparation in the craft of writing tests, so could you offer some guidelines for improving multiple-choice tests?*

DDP: Multiple-choice items require students to select the correct answer from an array of alternative responses written by the instructor. All multiple-choice items have the same three elements: The *stem* poses the question or presents a clinical scenario and the *key* is the correct answer or best option in a list of several *distractor* options that are likely to be plausible to a student who does not have a full grasp of the required knowledge. The following guidelines are culled from recommendations shared by measurement experts and experienced instructors.

1. Concentrate on writing items to *evaluate higher levels of thinking.* Avoid testing only memorization of basic factual knowledge.

2. Write the stem first.

3. *Concentrate on evaluating student ability to understand, apply, analyze, synthesize, and evaluate.* This is essential if you want to evaluate a student's critical thinking. Students have a tendency to study only "what will be on the test."

4. *State the problem or clinical scenario concisely and completely.* The student should be able to discern the problem *without* reading all of the options.

5. Write the stem to *include all the information essential to determining the question or the problem.* Omit irrelevant material that merely serves as padding, unless you want to test the student's determination of what is relevant.

6. *Avoid unnecessary repetition* by including as much of the item as possible in the stem.

7. *Ask the question in a positive form.* The use of negatives can be confusing to an anxious test taker. On rare occasions when you must use negatives, use **boldface**, <u>underlining</u>, or CAPITAL LETTERS. Do not use double negatives, for example, avoid negatives in both the stem and the options.

8. Write the correct or best response (key), after writing the stem. Be sure the best response is indeed *best*, as acknowledged in published text references and/or by authorities in the field.

9. Avoid making the key longer than the distractors.

10. Write the distractors after writing the key.

11. *Make all distractors plausible responses.* The effectiveness of multiple-choice items can be undermined by a sloppy preparation of distractors.

12. Write distractors that are distinct from each other.

13. Critique for general errors in style and format.

14. Be careful about using specific determiners, such as *all*, *never*, *always*, or other all-inclusive terms that are more likely to be found in incorrect options. Similarly, qualifiers such as *usually*, *sometimes*, and *maybe*, are more likely to be found in the keyed item.

15. *Avoid grammatical inconsistencies* between the stem and the options. These are very useful clues for the student who is competent in syntax.

16. Arrange options in a logical order. For example, numerical answers should be placed in ascending or descending numerical order; dates should be placed in chronological order.

Q: How can instructors best prepare students for exams? How can instructors help those students who freeze during exams?

DDP: An understanding of the process used to create the assessment helps tremendously. This reassures students who may be concerned about such things as trick questions, bias in grading, levels of difficulty, and the intent of the examination.

Instructors can do their utmost, but they cannot do the understanding *for* the student. During the test, the student has to draw on multiple resources to avoid freezing. This is not something that can be taught in a one-hour test preparation course. Students can turn to the beauty of their own medicine to diminish test anxiety, through acupressure or self-needling, centering through Tai Chi or Qigong, or drinking a relaxing (but not sleep inducing) tea.

It is important to acknowledge that just because a student scores high on a test, that does not necessarily equate with being the best practitioner.

5

Gained in Translation—Shiatsu and Trauma Workshops from Belfast to Vienna

PAMELA ELLEN FERGUSON, Dipl ABT (NCCAOM), AOBTA®-CI and GSD, LMT (Texas). *International Teacher of Shiatsu, former Director of Council of Schools and Programs, AOBTA®, and author of eight books (fiction and non fiction), including textbooks "The Self Shiatsu Handbook" (1) and "Take Five—The Five Elements Guide to Health and Harmony" (2)—published in English and German.*

Q: When you prepare to teach Trauma workshops for Continuing Education, how does your approach vary between Europe and the USA?

PEF: Whether it's Belfast, Berlin or Austin I start each class at a highly energetic pitch, lots of movement and paired stretching. This helps create a marvelous group energy, and more so when we are about to move into really deep and traumatic topics. Some of the groups in the German speaking countries are more accustomed to starting a class in a formal meditation circle. I don't, especially when dealing with Trauma. In any city I find that initiating a class in silence is too inhibiting, too isolating. Participants need to move, to interact, and to experience joy and fun in lively stretching exercises. Only then are they ready for silent *Qi* focusing.

Q: What else do you do to create a supportive environment?

PEF: I take a quick reading of the class dynamic, and get to know participants' names and professional experience in Shiatsu and related fields of medicine. I'm also very sensitive to the different ways in which people process trauma according to family or political context. I never use one individual's experience to define a group, and never force anything.

It's probably easier for me to be experimental and adventurous in my global workshops because I've lived in Europe, North America, Africa and the Middle East. I've experienced civil war, states-of-emergency, tear gas, cancer, family suicides, cycling accidents, tornadoes and hurricanes, and have always taken incredible risks. During my years as a journalist I've interviewed former political prisoners who've survived torture. So my students know I adapt Shiatsu through the crucible of experience and not through someone else's "textbook" theory.

Participants are all Shiatsu Therapists, and many are also Physical Therapists, RNs, Acupuncturists and Psychologists. Many often start sharing their own personal traumas—not just the traumas of patients who are survivors of wars, political torture, domestic or urban violence, and various accidents. Taboo topics often crop up like physical or emotional trauma in marriage. Some discuss experiences like spousal rape during pregnancy. Others describe flashbacks they experienced while giving birth, when memories surfaced of sexual abuse during childhood.

I encourage everyone to utilize personal experiences—not to share with patients of course—but to help deepen diagnostic insights and creative treatments.

Q: How do you structure the Trauma workshops?

PEF: During the first hour I teach treatment procedures for whiplash to anchor the class within a safe structure. Everybody can relate to whiplash. So we strike a common chord. To address the source problem we perform very simple off-the-body exercises around the patient's head to repair "fragmented *Qi*," using the image of pieces of fragmented glass coming together in a perfect mirror or plate glass window, as in a TV action replay. This is vital before selective meridians and points can be treated. Then we discuss simple ways of recognizing and treating whiplash spin-offs, like headaches, vertigo, chronic neck pain, fear, insomnia, problems with swallowing and so on. We also discuss the extreme sensitivity of the neck area and ways in which head, neck and jaw can be a depository for many levels of trauma, not just whiplash, and how memories can be triggered when you simply support the neck with sensitivity.

Following whiplash, we move logically towards the "road accident" as a basic model. I ask any one of the participants to run us through the details of some personal experience of an auto or bicycle accident. Initially we co-create a Five Element profile of the accident on the flip chart (season, road conditions, time of day, purpose of journey, etc.) and then re-create the actual accident on a large sheet of drawing paper on the floor, using colorful markers, stickers, and matchbox cars, trucks and bicycles. This not only helps the participant to objectify the accident in a colorful way, but it prompts memory in terms of the physics of the accident and can help explain a bizarre range of injuries and any form of Post Traumatic Stress Disorder (fear of crossroads, fear of driving in mist, bouts of depression, etc.). We can then relate those injuries and fears to specific meridians and acupoints, and add new diagnostic insights to the Five Element profile.

I then encourage all participants to pair up and externalize some past accident or trauma from their own lives, using large drawing pads, pens, stickers of people of all races, flowers, animals, stars and hearts. They hunker down like kids and love the exercise.

Q: How do you relate the drawings to Shiatsu?

PEF: I discuss each drawing individually and encourage each pair of participants to make diagnostic assessments of those drawings in discussions with one another in terms of the Five Elements, meridians and points, and then to treat one another with the specific purpose of healing any lingering or unresolved emotional or physical scar prompted by the incident. Interestingly enough, the spontaneous pairing of participants often brought people with similar experiences together, or experiences that complemented or deepened a special insight or understanding of the context of the incident and any resulting spin-offs. The exercise is simple, colorful, can be humorous, and helps participants develop new diagnostic and treatment procedures that can be applied to more complex situations for their patients.

One participant reconstructed a cycling accident that killed her husband some 20 years prior when she was pregnant with their first child. Using stickers of tiny red hearts, she linked a figure she drew of her pregnant self, with the figure she drew of her fatally injured husband. After his death, she was not permitted to see his body because of the damage, so in some ways she never achieved a sense of closure. She experienced a new level of healing and clarity through this exercise that extended through the compassionate Shiatsu session she received from her work partner.

Q: How do the responses to trauma differ between nationalities?

PEF: Usually, American, Canadian, Italian, and Spanish participants find it somewhat easier to share traumatic experiences from their lives. German, Irish, Swiss, Dutch, British, or Austrian participants tend to share trauma bit by bit, in layers that feel safe for them. And second generation Asians in Europe or North America tend to find it easier than their parents or grandparents to talk about trauma. A Vietnamese American student sought my treatment advice for her parents who were devastated by the Hurricane Katrina disaster in the USA in 2005. I said "But this is a double trauma. Weren't your parents Boat People from Vietnam?" "Oh yes!" she said, "but that's taboo. We don't talk about that."

Q: How do the accident reconstructions in your workshops prompt deeper sharings?

PEF: I never force anything in my classes and the last thing we encourage is some group catharsis. But on Day Two of my workshops, women and men often begin to share deeper experiences, and quite spontaneously so. This is where the "whiplash" component offers such a safe foundation. The following stories emerged in workshops from Belfast to Hamburg, from Amsterdam to Zurich, from Berlin to Vienna. To mention a few, with pseudonyms, Nelly spoke about the neck damage she experienced when her mother gave birth to her, resulting in neck tremors when she entered adolescence and difficulties when she gave birth to her own kids. Brigid spoke about the trauma she experienced in a foreign city when a doctor tried to molest her one night after she was hospitalized and immobilized by a neck brace and leg plaster following an auto accident. Freddie spoke about the brutality of a father who beat him constantly for no reason. Trudy described the trauma of her husband's rage after she survived an auto accident that damaged his fancy car. Maria, who is also an Egyptologist, witnessed the terrorist attack on a group of tourists in Luxor, Egypt. Being multilingual, she helped survivors and the rescue crew, but underestimated the emotional impact on herself, and found it hard to justify until our workshop.

There were shades of differences in how each individual processed the trauma—not necessarily according to cultural backgrounds—but according to whether individuals—or their parents—also experienced war or civil war, or whether they were in a hometown or foreign country, and especially, whether they had supportive or dismissive families and relationships. A sense of isolation within or following a trauma can compound the effects—and resulting PTSD—for years. Similarly, intergenerational trauma plays a big role in the lives of those who were raised by parents who experienced severe war trauma. One participant spoke about his lifelong battles with depression because his father collaborated with a fascist regime.

Q: How do participants share their stories in layers?

PEF: Here's a stark example. Carla drew a picture on Day One of an experience she had with an indifferent Tai Chi teacher in China who stood by and did nothing to help her during a class when she injured herself. He told her dismissively that the injury was all "part of the work." I could tell from Carla's expression and distress that this story was layered over something far more traumatic. Spontaneously on Day Two, she told us how her enraged husband tried to murder her one night by snapping her neck, and how she broke his hold using a Tai Chi movement, and how she ran into the night and traveled hours by cab to a close friend. The connecting link between the stories was not only Tai Chi, but an authority figure being dismissive. The police disregarded her charge against her husband, saying "nothing happened." And her mother's first question was, "what did you do to enrage your husband?" Interestingly, Carla continues to teach Tai Chi to this day as part of her ongoing path to healing.

Q: How do participants in your workshops gravitate toward other participants with shared experiences?

PEF: Some bond with others who share experiences of political—or religious—oppression—even at opposite ends of the globe! For example two participants—both experienced Shiatsu therapists and mothers in their 40s—gravitated towards one another on a deep level and spontaneously so, only to discover that each shared very different but abusive sexual experiences as children from people associated with their Roman Catholic church. They grew up in different parts of the world, had very different family backgrounds, spoke different languages, but this particular bond was immediate, profound, and powerful. Both began to relate subsequent traumas and emotional challenges as adults to those early experiences.

Q: Aren't subtleties lost in translation when you deal with these emotionally charged topics in different cities?

PEF: Quite the contrary. Sometimes I think people open up more when the teacher is from another country, and the translation process can provide a sort of "buffer." Working with a German translator requires short, clear, crisp sentences in English, because the German translation is often much longer, and it's important to keep up the momentum. People who are bilingual hear everything in both languages, and they like that. Sometimes certain facts or discussions are more acceptable in a foreign language. So the translation process has a balancing effect. My workshops have been translated into German, Swiss German, French, Spanish, Romansch, Lithuanian, and Xhosa. When it's German or French, I know enough in both languages to pick up on a misunderstanding or mistranslation, and then the word becomes a matter of group discussion and often a useful teaching point. We are quick to spot humor even in the darkest moments. I maximize those moments especially when funny misunderstandings arise around mistranslations, like the time "dry vagina" was translated as "drive to China" in a class in Switzerland on menopause. Everyone laughed so hard I had to call a break—but they remembered everything they learned that day because of the laughter. In another workshop people looked baffled when I taught *Qi* exercises according to compass directions, because "compass" was translated as "compost". I heard of another teacher who didn't realize that his constant reference to "life forces" was being translated as "live horses" until someone in the class figured it out.

Q: What general national or cultural differences do you observe and respond to as a teacher?

PEF: I don't want to make sweeping generalizations, but I've noticed that when we do role-playing for an insight into, say, body language, or characteristics or reactions we have observed in patients, as a way of *experiencing* the specific physical/or specific meridian distortion, American, Canadian, Spanish, Russian and Italian participants have no problem with the exercise. They love to role play, and it's always hard to stop them! But many German participants freeze, wary of "taking on" the characteristics and the problems until I convince them that this is pure theatre—nothing more—and show them how to protect themselves by imagining themselves in a protective "bubble of *Qi*." Swiss participants start off a little wary, and need convincing, but Zurich is nowhere near as hard to convince as Berlin!

On the flip side, American students learn very well with their eyes (probably because of so much TV) but not all of them take notes, and many ask for printed handouts and/or videos. Certainly they are accustomed to more spoon feeding. My students in Germany, Switzerland and Austria never, ever ask for printed handouts or videos, and they are all, to a person, excellent and copious note-takers. Their notebooks are works of art, a teacher's dream, often dotted with little stick figures depicting exercises and treatment positions. However, I often have to remind them to put down their notebooks and *watch* what I am demonstrating. In America it's the other way around, I have to encourage many of them to take notes! Canadian students (English and French speaking) hover midway between their American and European counterparts. They watch *and* take excellent notes.

In Europe I also have to be very tactful when giving advice about the specific Shiatsu techniques participants may have been taught in their basic training but should avoid when working with trauma, like sitting too close to patients, shaking or rocking patients, or leaning over them. Encouraging participants to modify body mechanics for this highly specialized Shiatsu often requires more explanation in the German speaking countries, than perhaps it might take in the USA or Canada where participants have certainly experienced a less authoritarian school system.

Q: *What other treatment guidelines do you teach in Trauma workshops?*

PEF: For Trauma and PTSD patients, generally, I also advise a simple, linear and very structured form of Shiatsu, clearly defined and direct, and well explained. Minimalism is the key. Less is more. No invasive or forceful techniques at all. But I also teach everyone how to recognize symptoms of trauma in patients who may come for any number of other reasons, back pain, headaches, stress or whatever. Sudden physical reactions, twisting, pulling away, startled moves, can all convey some unresolved trauma. UB 23 (Kidney-Back Shu/Yu Point) in particular seems to hold a memory bank of past trauma, as does the Kidney Meridian. So I always advise everyone to be extra observant around these areas, similarly, to be extra sensitive when working on meridians in vulnerable zones: inner thigh, sacrum, umbilicus and so on. Stretching can also prompt memories. I prepare everyone to remain calm and centered, even when/if a patient reacts or suddenly pulls away. We also discuss referral options in situations where a patient clearly needs professional counseling beyond the scope of practice of Shiatsu.

Q: *Would you like to share some case studies?*

PEF: A patient came to me in the USA for fibromyalgia, "When did it start?" I asked. "Four years ago," she replied. "What happened four years ago?" She was in a road accident, she explained, but her doctors told her there was no connection. "Oh?" I said, and suggested we reconstruct the accident on a drawing pad. Then she shared the details. She was at the wheel, they were hit head on by a drunk driver, and her husband was thrown from the car and killed. And yes, she felt a mixture of guilt, grief, and anger, all of which had literally locked down her Gall Bladder meridian. After one Shiatsu session she experienced a marked reduction in pain, which continued after she took my advice and joined a Qigong class. If I had just treated the woman's fibromyalgia she would probably still be coming for sessions. Instead, she came for one session, and later returned to share the story of her experience with my students.

In one of my clinic theater classes I invited a guy who had nearly lost his life on a train dynamited by some extremist group in a Latin American country. He experienced considerable muscle and tissue damage and had reconstructive surgery on his arms and legs. He felt comfortable sharing the experience surrounded by my students. I supported his hand and wrist to be able to feel the reactions in his *Qi* as he related the incident. I discovered deeply traumatized Kidney and San Jiao meridians. But the experience of being with us helped him put the incident into a new framework, especially when I advised him to return to the area of the attack at some safe time in the future, and complete the journey that had been shattered.

Q: *As you have personally experienced war, are you working with war damaged members of the military experiencing PTSD?*

PEF: I am working with Shiatsu colleagues who are associated with the military, and am in discussion with other therapists who are treating complex cases of PTSD. This is a highly controversial area as many cases are being dealt with inadequately by the military, according to media reports (3). I am encouraging the deeper involvement of Shiatsu in long term PTSD care.

Q: What self-care do you practice when teaching Trauma workshops in your compressed international schedule?

PEF: I spend hours replenishing while traveling by train through glorious landscapes between cities in Europe. I walk for hours along the Rhine in Basel or Heidelberg, or along the Elbe in Dresden or beside the lake of Zurich or along the canals in Berlin or Amsterdam. I take photographs of bicycles in every possible context. I also spend hours in art museums in the cities where I teach. And in my workshops I love sharing examples of painters like Frida Kahlo, Edvard Munch, Vincent van Gogh, and Rene Magritte—all of whom transformed their individual experiences of trauma into incredible art.

6

Shiatsu and Counseling in Zurich

MADINA BOKOUM *is certified by the Swiss Shiatsu Society (SGS—Dipl. Shiat-supraktikerin) and is a certified counselor (Psychologische Beratung) and combines both qualifications in her practice in Zurich and Bern Switzerland. Part Swiss and part West African, Madina was raised in Basel and educated in France and Switzerland. She is a co-founder of Flying Ki Shiatsu School, Zurich, to create experimental Continuing Education workshops for Shiatsu Therapists, many of whom are also Physical Therapists, RNs and Psychologists.*

Q: *How do you advise your patients and students to avoid Burnout?*

MB: I try to figure out how they take breaks. It's hard to tell the Swiss to take breaks—many have been raised believing, "fun is not good." One of the most important questions I ask them is, what are you rushing for? What triggers this rushing? What is your goal? Do you have financial troubles? We try to work out the answers and new directions together and with a lot of humor. I also ask them, what is the critical time in the day for you? OK, show me that peak moment of high stress. Show me *physically*. I ask them to emphasize the posture—then they recognize the stress pattern immediately—and some even fall over. Then I do physical exercises to ground them. I teach their bodies to get grounded. This helps them let go. The feeling is good and they think, hey, that's the sensation I'd like to experience more often. I try to work on prevention when I fear upcoming burnout.

Q: *Describe the supervision/counseling you give to Shiatsu Therapists in Switzerland as part of their future Continuing Education requirements to renew their annual membership in the Swiss Shiatsu*

Society? You are one of the few Continuing Education providers qualified to do this specialized supervision.

MB: There's no simple recipe for this supervision/counseling, but I'll share just one example among a million possible examples and approaches. Therapists can choose to consult me on their own, or in a group of other colleagues, to discuss psychosocial problems, that could relate to their interactions with a patient, or with a colleague, or may reflect something more personal.

Let's say they come to me with a problem they have interacting with an anorectic patient. Then I ask, why do you have a problem? The problem is the patient's—not yours! Basically I want to know why the therapist has a problem relating to anorexia. Then I do an exercise with them—a self empowerment exercise—I ask them to go into the exact situation when the patient stressed them—it might be a sentence, a word, a gesture, or the way the patient lies down. I want to know—what is there that makes the therapist feel uncomfortable?

Then I ask them to describe how they feel. Maybe they feel nausea. Then I say, let's imagine your best friend is in the room—what should he/she do for you in this moment? What kind of input would be helpful? So they come up with a solution.

Then I ask them—how does this feel now? This often prompts an awareness of the source of the problem. And it's OK if they become aware of the source problem. This could be a fear of their own anorexia or the death of a friend from anorexia. I say—give this fear the space it needs.... but know it has space.... be aware of it or it dances around....

Eventually I want to create a space where they can explore their problem. Therapists have to recognize that there is a problem. Once they recognize it they talk differently and act differently around that patient. If there is no improvement they need to refer the patient to an appropriate colleague.

Other therapists may come to me with a problem relating to a patient who is terminally ill, or battling addiction, or going through a separation. Dealing with different problems requires great flexibility and a global view.

I may start a supervision/counseling session with a therapist with one intention in mind until I realize that a whole other technique may be more appropriate. So I switch techniques. As I say there can be a million ways of working with supervision/counseling.

Q: *What are the benefits of this type of supervision, and do you feel there is sufficient basic training in psychosocial aspects of therapy in the Shiatsu curriculum?*

MB: Benefits? It makes the work more interesting! You don't get burnt out, or fall into a routine—because the therapist is learning a lot about him/herself and is evolving through this. And no—there isn't sufficient psychosocial training in the basic Shiatsu curriculum. Most Shiatsu instructors don't have the advanced education required to deal with such topics—even if they sometimes think they do!

Q: *In one of your workshops you mentioned the case of a patient who came to you for headaches—and after five sessions with barely any change, you realized the problem was deeper. You shared your sense of impasse with her. As a result she opened up to you and shared her acute distress because her teenage son was abusing her teenage daughter sexually. What helped her to open up to you and share a deep taboo?*

MB: Sometimes if I reach an impasse with a patient I will share this with them and say, I'm lost. I don't understand. I don't know what to do. Help me here. And in this case the woman shared her pain. Now, the Swiss aren't generally good at communicating. The French are much more open about discussing taboos. The Swiss think it's "not polite" to discuss certain topics. This particular patient hadn't even been able to discuss the problem with her husband, but she shared it with me. I told her she needed help, she couldn't deal with the problem on her own, and I planned to follow through with more advice in future sessions. The headache vanished while we were talking. But I never saw her again.

Q: *Most Shiatsu Therapists do not have your training in psychology/counseling. What advice do you give them when patients share problems that require more than basic Shiatsu, as in the above case?*

MB: Acknowledge the patients' courage and openness. Don't try to save your patients. Don't treat them like ill people or like children. Shiatsu Therapists need to know when to refer—immediately—and not attempt to handle a complex problem like this unless they have had special training. But all Shiatsu Therapists just need to be open to the problems patients share quite spontaneously, and ask the patient, have you looked for help? Or is there a reason why you haven't? Can I refer you to a colleague? It's very important to acknowledge whatever the patient has tried to do so far.

Q: Two of your patients committed suicide during one year of your practice. As a therapist, how do you cope with such realities? And what guidelines do you give other therapists to help them with suicidal patients?

MB: I take a very practical view. My Shiatsu practice is not the place where patients who are in acute danger can be treated. There are psychiatric clinics for that. My particular patients had deep depressions but I was only able to refer one of them to a clinic. The other patient refused further treatment and was "happy" to enjoy Shiatsu as it relieved his chronic insomnia. But in both cases my patients just wanted Shiatsu like a quick fix and didn't want to change anything in their lives—and they blocked the therapy.

There was a third suicide case involving the father of one of my patients, who I did not know personally. That suicide happened a couple of days after I had treated his son and I had a strong feeling that something serious was going on in the family. Such work is very complex. Shiatsu Therapists should always refer suicidal patients to hotlines or psychiatrists.

Q: Your workshops involve an exercise where participants pair up, one stands still and the other walks towards/her/him to test boundary issues. Some participants held their partners at arms' length. Others just stood there and let their partners crash into them physically. What do participants learn from this exercise?

MB: They learn about boundary issues—how they set/or do not set boundaries and this can be very surprising—I've known very strong people who let their partner crash into them—and were afraid to see this. But they had to feel it physically. Then I work with them and reverse the roles, to see how they feel when others stop them, or how they stop them (with hands raised, or with a gesture, or a glance, or a sound.) The question is this, how do you create your own space? What is your own space and how do you define it?

Q: Your experimental workshop "Nicht Bei Uns" ("Not Amongst/With Us") explores the effect of a number of taboos on health, namely, racism, sexism, emotional/and/or physical abuse in marriage, and bullying in the workplace or at school. Do you feel such taboos go largely unrecognized in mainstream medicine in Switzerland? How can Shiatsu help?

MB: Yes, such problems are largely unrecognized in mainstream medicine. Shiatsu helps because patients have a full hour with the practitioner and not just 10 minutes, and have close contact with a practitioner, which they don't have with doctors. But again, many Swiss patients feel uncomfortable about sharing these problems because they consider this "impolite." And when they do share such experiences, Shiatsu alone is often not enough, even though it can provide the first moment where a patient feels comfortable about discussing a personal problem. And Shiatsu is so helpful when patients seem to have lost contact with themselves and when they get "stuck."

Q: How accessible is Shiatsu in Switzerland?

MB: Shiatsu is very well integrated in the Swiss health system. It's covered by health insurance, without a doctor's prescription, but therapists must belong to the Swiss Shiatsu Society, which means that they have been fully trained for at least three years and attend continuing education workshops every year. Some health insurance companies would only raise a question if they noticed no change in a patient's condition after, say, ten sessions.

Q: As you grew up bi-racial in Switzerland, and were educated in France, have you always had a rare insight as an insider/outsider where many people assume you aren't Swiss? And how has this helped your evolution as a therapist, and your own rare ability to work with patients from a wide cross section of cultural and ethnic backgrounds?

MB: Ninety percent of my patients are Swiss, but most of them have lived or worked internationally, and maybe half of them are married to/or in relationships with a foreigner. And there I probably am more helpful than I actually realize. Foreigners do not scare me in the way they may scare some Swiss people. I also tell my patients to acknowledge the fact that it is much more difficult to *really* understand a foreign culture than we actually think.

Q: Can you give some examples of the cross cultural differences you come across in your clinical practice?

MB: Patients who can't deal with other cultures, probably come to me only once. The cross mix of patients I have treated include people from cultures where they only feel their bodies through pain—especially women from certain Middle Eastern countries. And for some people, the whole issue of psychosomatic symptoms does not exist and they just come to Shiatsu for a quick-fix—especially some people from Eastern Europe on a fast track business career.

Q: How do you teach your students (who may not have the same background in counseling as you) to help their patients prepare for death?

MB: I'd ask them to see for themselves how they deal with death based on their own experiences. If they have never dealt with death and are afraid of it, then I suggest they seek help for themselves from a more experienced specialized therapist. We have many different workshops on death/mourning in Switzerland, ranging from the Elisabeth Kübler-Ross approach, to the rituals of classical Greece. In the healing profession, sooner or later you have to deal with death. I personally often have patients in my practice who experienced a family death or death of someone close in the previous couple of months.

Q: Switzerland is a tiny country, but is famous for producing some rare and pioneering physicians like Albert Schweitzer, Carl Jung, and Elisabeth Kübler-Ross. Why do you think this is?

MB: For me this was normal, I've never been asked this question before. Switzerland has always had a high profile as a haven of healing, mainly because of the mountains, the clean air, and hospitals or sanatoria in beautiful settings—something we take for granted. Ask me why Zurich seems to have more psychologists than most cities? I can't answer that. Is it because Switzerland has one of the highest standards of living? But because Switzerland wasn't invaded during World War I and World War II, Swiss medical teams have always moved around the globe with organizations like the Red Cross to work within war damaged countries. Maybe all of this has inspired pioneers in medicine?

7

Teachers We've All Known—the Best and the Rest

DEBRA C. HOWARD, Dipl ABT (NCCAOM), AOBTA®-CI, LMT *was AOBTA President from 2002–2007 and currently serves on the faculty at Medical Training College in Baton Rouge, Louisiana. Debra taught at the Blue Cliff School of Therapeutic Massage in New Orleans for seven years. She has authored introductory chapters on ABT and Shiatsu in "Massage Therapy Principles and Practice" (1) and in "Introduction to Massage Therapy" (2)*

Q: I heard you say one of the main reasons you became an instructor was because of your dismay at some of the poor instruction you experienced during your own training. True? Can you elaborate?

DH: Yes, it's true.... and not only in my ABT and MT training, though that is where my own teaching intent really bloomed. I'm pretty sure I've always had an opinion (well—what can I say?) about what learning is, what's worth learning in a classroom environment, and how it is best facilitated. Even in early grade school, I remember thinking that I wished they would teach me more I could really use, in a way that I could understand, so I would know how to use the knowledge in a practical way. I loved the teachers who could do that for me! I've had some good teachers and I've had some who drove me nuts—and some who were a little nutty, but that was OK with me. I realize that what qualifies as a 'good teacher' can be very subjective, but I also think certain things are necessary for a teacher to really be 'good'. I guess what qualifies me to say anything about it at all is that I love to learn! I enjoy being a student with a good teacher. My best teachers have been those who truly loved what they were doing. They were not only learned, they were experienced in their subject(s).

The best teachers:

- Offered their knowledge freely;
- Didn't play power games in class;
- Didn't look down on the class as 'lowly students'; treated students with respect and conducted the classes in a relaxed, yet professional, manner;
- Had humor to share, and enjoyed interacting with students and helping us learn;
- Had clear syllabi, lesson plans, tests, boundaries, and expectations in class;
- Didn't run scared from, or overreact to, problem students;
- Left plenty of room for *fun*;
- Gave clear explanations to students;
- Were fair and consistent across the board;
- Provided a good bridge between students and the school administration; and
- Offered the best of what they had.

Some of the worst teachers:

- Didn't teach the subject (*oh, sorry—what were we here for?*);
- Read from a textbook through the entire class (*sssnnnnzzzgh*);
- Played ego games and had power struggles with students (*I said we're going to do it my way!*);
- Arrived unprepared for class (*I forgot to make the handout copies, and what day are we ending again?*);
- Did not allow enough time to assimilate material by throwing out too much at once—or by combining topics that were impossible to follow (*Class One, Day Two: so then it's this, unless that is happening, or that, or unless this minor possibility pops up—or not …*);
- Did not care if students actually understood the material (*I presented the material, so what's the problem?*);
- Let unruly students disrupt the whole class (*'I wish the teacher would tell those guys to be quiet or get out'*);

- Let unethical students continue without confrontation (*if I don't report them, they won't hate me, or retaliate*);
- Played 'serious games'—like the teacher who locked us out of the class-room and wouldn't let us in until exactly 9am; and
- Played "mystical" games, like the instructor who attempted to put our entire class into a trance without first addressing what was being done and asking permission (*and now, let yourself be totally relaxed and listen only to my voice....*).

There were also teachers whom I really liked as people, but were still not good teachers. They had good intentions, but were often too scattered and too loose in their class structure, or too 'personal' (focused on personal issues) for my learning tastes. There were others who offered too much of themselves and burnt out. And of course, there were those I disliked as people, but were wonderful teachers. And of course there's a lot to be said for multiple layers of challenges in a learning environment.

Teachers who have to be friends with all the students are not my favor-ite—they often make educational and institutional mistakes because they want to be liked more than to focus on education. If teachers are too aloof and unap-proachable, students will not even attempt to connect. I think mutual respect is a better relationship for teaching; a somewhat strict approach with clear protocols alleviates favoritism.

Q: What additional advice would you give to a bright, eager ABT graduate about becoming an instructor?

DH: I would probably suggest they itemize the things they admire and respect about their best/favorite teachers, and see if they can incorporate those qualities in their own teaching styles. For comparison, it's equally good to itemize the things they like the least about instructors they've had, and avoid those qualities in their teaching.

Q: What is the best way to train Instructors?

DH: Assistant teaching! Make sure they are involved with every level of teaching experience, from taking roll to filling out grade sheets; from counseling a student who is failing, or problematic, to honoring a student who is outstanding, and from working directly with the school administration to congratulating proud parents.

There is also much that can be learned through teacher-training classes and class materials. I find it very helpful to hear of others' experiences and to ask advice of those who might be able to help me. Differing learning styles can be taught verbally, but the value of direct experience using that knowledge in class cannot be understated.

Interpersonal boundaries with school administration, other faculty, school staff, students and other interested parties are a worthy topic of discussion and practice for a budding teacher. If they are naturally gifted teachers, don't mess with them too much. You don't want to ruin them! In my opinion, seeing yourself teach on videotape is also invaluable training (*Oh, dear! Do I really touch my nose like that—and that often?*).

Q: How does the curriculum you created differ from the curriculum you experienced in your own training?

DH: I created a new curriculum several years ago at another school and took more time to teach the material. I thought what I was originally taught in 150 hours would take at least 300 hours to teach. I was right about that—in fact, now I would say even more time is necessary. ABT, in particular, is learning about life anew! Learning a new way to think while also learning a new language, and new philosophies, tends to take a while longer than learning a new technique. I now think that training an Asian Bodywork Therapy practitioner successfully in the USA requires a minimum two-year program, especially if the practitioner wishes to have a successful private practice.

My approaches are different from my personal experiences as an ABT student:

- I offer students clear handouts that I have created, targeted homework assignments, and study guides.
- I work to keep the material as clear and concise as possible.
- Even though Chinese Medicine and ABT are circular and cyclical in nature, we have to find a way to teach it in a linear fashion, since this is how we experience time. This has been a big challenge.

- Keeping in as much experiential activity as possible is a must, to avoid a long lecture. (*oh, man, I can talk sometimes!*)

- I demonstrate and then the students trade with each other while I work along with them. We rotate around the room while practicing techniques.

- We stretch, move, and breathe every day—sometimes more than once!

- Stretching in pairs, or group Bodywork in a line or circle is always fun for students and builds unity in the classroom.

I love to take the class outside, especially if it's a beautiful day, so we can experience the wholism and natural base of what we are learning. The medical theory can be applied much better if it can also be related to something students can see in nature right before them. There are many different aspects of the training that I approach on a very practical level. Along with lots of practice of ABT assessment and treatment skills, we cook and eat balanced meals while we're studying food energetics; practice Moxibustion, Cupping, and Guasha when studying adjunct therapies; practice Qigong and other *Qi* experiences daily; share case studies, clinic experiences, and personal development issues. We also have supervised study groups in, and out of class.

We review material in class (a lot!). We go through tests together so students can see their mistakes and ask questions. Students trade assessments and treatments, and evaluate each other (draw numbers for partners, and ask for honest feedback—see what happens!).

I highly recommend students receive sessions from two or three professional ABTs in the area, to see how those treatments affect their perception of ABT, and how they compare with their own homework treatment sessions. I make myself available to students as needed and as appropriate.

Q: *What is the best way for schools to test a student's practical, clinical, and theoretical skills?*

DH: This is the $64,000 question, isn't it? Without ways to measure a student's practical skills and theoretical knowledge, how do we determine their success and support their subsequent graduation, certification, licensure, and practice?

Schools have an obligation to weed out those who truly cannot do this work, or are unethical, violent, or otherwise unsuitable for professional practice. Each school determines their boundaries in this area. Teachers are the gatekeepers. Unfortunately, some of my experiences have shown it's more valuable for the school to keep the students in, let them graduate, and "let nature take its course" in determining their fate. This 'natural course' can have a devastating effect on an emerging profession, not to mention the time and effort wasted by the student and everyone else at the school.

The ideal way of testing <u>practical skills at the school/program level</u> is for the student to:

- Provide a session or perform specific techniques on an instructor, or an experienced practitioner. Clear guidelines on what is being tested, and a clear grading scale, will prevent much of the subjectivity of the past (i.e., it's not enough to say *I didn't like it,* and give a low or failing grade).

<u>Student Clinic</u> skills are generally best tested in three ways, with:

- Clearly outlined goals set by the supervising instructor, who will grade students in a clearly defined way.
- Written and verbal feedback from the clients, post-session.
- Self-grading by the students, who are often surprisingly harsh on themselves.

<u>Theoretical</u> skills are generally best tested with a viable paper or computer test. You can test a 'classic example' of theory in a written form, but when it comes to using that information on real clients, supervised clinical practice, or internship/apprenticeship, is a better measure.

Q: *What about testing at a national level for professional certification?*

DH: The multiple-choice exam format is pretty awful, in my opinion, but the best we have at present. Students can almost 'guess' their way through a multiple-choice test. I think this format was adopted because it is 'easily' created and graded, is considered fair to all students, and is reasonably cost-efficient. Unfortunately, a lot of the power and credibility of testing is lost, due to the 'guess factor'. Don't get me wrong, I think national certification is wonderful! I just wish the system worked differently.

Q: How do you help students overcome examination nerves?

DH: I generally start by asking them what is the worst that can happen?—then we discuss what it might mean if they fail. We look at test-taking strategies, the how and why of testing anyway, and strengthen their knowledge of testing in general.

Other tips:

- Use Qigong, breathing techniques, acupressure, and other stress-relieving techniques you know. It's a great opportunity to show them how ABT can help them when they learn how to use it!

- Practice with a test that's entirely ridiculous. They can experience a failure, then move past it. Tie that in with the training, discussing assessment and treatment of this imbalance.

- Discuss teas and useful homeopathic remedies.

- Discuss study tactics and memory methods—like eating the same food before you test as you eat when you study! Yum. Look at foods to enjoy, and foods to avoid.

- We also review class material many times over. Sometimes the confidence of being well prepared is enough to overcome the anxiety.

Q: How do you deal with problem students?

DH: It depends on the nature of the problem. The bottom line? Mutual respect has been the best avenue for me. I prefer to be as direct and clear as possible, without any glossing-over of the issues, and to outline clearly what has happened, what is expected, and how the issues can be resolved. Including a timeline is very helpful. An 'under-emotional' approach has worked best for me. Too much emotion and you lose the message.

It's also very important to be open to hearing what the student has to say. I like to learn all the students' names the very first day. Especially the 'problem children' … they're easy to spot within the first few minutes of class, so I like to engage them directly—and quickly. The students like my interest in them and that I can identify each of them at the end of the first class. It's also a 'heads-up' for them. I know who they are and though I want to have fun, we are also here to meet certain goals.

Q: How do you adapt your teaching to meet the needs of increasingly varied groups of students, of all ages, backgrounds, professions, and learning skills?

DH: It's challenging! I use as many different media and different approaches as I can. Transparencies, paper handouts, video presentations, books and other reading material, audiotapes—anything, really, that seems interesting and serves a purpose in our training.

Also:

- Use a variety of materials to help with varied learning styles.

- Lots of Bodywork practice helps, allowing time for students to explore what they are doing 'on their own' (stay nearby to respond to questions).

- Tie the theory in with the practice as often, and in as many ways, as possible.

- Creative projects are an invaluable tool. Students learn by creating their projects, and learn from other students' projects.

- It's helpful to teach mostly to the mid-to-upper-academic-level students, and ask them to help others in the class who are having trouble. If you focus too much on those who are struggling, you may lose the ones who may be truly gifted. In addition, those who help teach the others gain valuable new skills, too.

Q: How has your own teaching method evolved over the past few years?

DH: My teaching methods are (hopefully) always changing in response to the environment in which I'm teaching and my own personal development. In general, I find that I talk faster to keep the younger students' attention, moving from subject to subject or task to task more quickly. They have no abilities to focus for long periods of time (modern life is overstimulating!).

I use many tried and true methods that haven't changed much over the past few years:

- Start with the big picture and work into the smaller focus;
- Offer smaller bits of new material at a time;

- Repeat the stuff that has to be memorized—over and over and over;

- In order to keep myself interested, I work with bare bones materials—meaning I don't use a lot of notes. This sparks my creativity and understanding; and

- I do my best to use different ways to explain things each time we review.

8

Back from Burnout in Britain

CAROLA BERESFORD-COOKE, BA, LicAc, MRSS, *British based Acupuncturist and International Teacher of Shiatsu, and author of a major textbook "Shiatsu Theory and Practice" (1) published in English and German.*

Q: What are the warning signs of burnout for practitioners and instructors?

CBC: I would say for both a reluctance to engage in the practice, a feeling of dread or inadequacy, dissatisfaction afterwards and a slowness to recover. Not enjoying it, to be precise. And signs of depression—poor sleep, inability to relax, excessive fatigue, negative outlook.

Q: How do you advise students to avoid burnout?

CBC: We teach them not to invest themselves in the outcome of treatment, to relax physically. But burnout usually comes further down the line and there are other dragons to overcome first. I did once warn a student I was assessing that if she kept on over-extending her energy she would burn out quite soon, but I doubt if she took any notice. It is all so exciting to start with, and we are so into *doing*!

Q: How do you advise your colleagues to avoid burnout?

CBC: Stop working, or radically curtail working, and rest. Take a holiday. Or, find another profession altogether.

Q: How do you prevent burnout?

CBC: I would not have taken on having a child at 45, a move to the country, an exhausting rural domestic schedule, learning Welsh, editing the Shiatsu Society Newsletter, etc … And of course I would have avoided menopause.…

Q: And your solution?

CBC: Sit and stare … actually what is ideal for me is an uncluttered horizon—a day I can drift through at my own rhythm, with nobody wanting me to do anything and no deadlines.

Q: Has your crafting of the third edition of "Shiatsu Theory and Practice" helped to energize you out of your burnout?

CBC: Not exactly, in fact I would say it is the other way around. Having taken time out to rest and slowly to begin to enjoy the rest of my life, I find it is all now feeding back into my work.

All the aspects of my life that seemed so burdensome, the rural domestic schedule, the care for my family, have become sources of joy and insight as I have had time to engage in them fully. That joy has entered into my treatments, which in turn have also provided new material for reflection.

Q: Do you advise colleagues to explore writing or other creative exercises as a way out of the labyrinth of burnout?

CBC: I am sure that it is appropriate for many people to do so, but I would never advise anyone suffering from burnout to do anything but rest and allow their inner self to recover to the point where it can guide them once more.

Q: You said your third edition has inspired you to "start from scratch." Do you feel burnout enabled you to have the necessary distance and retreat to help you re-tool?

CBC: Absolutely!

Q: Or, has extensive feedback from students and instructors inspired you to tackle the work anew?

CBC: I wish I could say I'd been inspired by something, but in fact it is an imperative from my publishers that is propelling me forwards! I would personally have liked a couple more years doing very little before engaging with the task.

Q: Your impressive analyses of the traditional meridians compared with the Masunaga extended meridians have prompted some scepticism among colleagues who practise only Shiatsu, but praise and appreciation among colleagues who practise both Acupuncture and Shiatsu. Thoughts?

CBC: Well, it's interesting that it's that way round; but scepticism is all right by me. Whatever model of the human energy system is proposed it will never come close to the amazing reality of our existence. What I mean is really, systems, shmystems, just get your hands on.

9

Quotes on Burnout from Around the World

I'm not a workaholic. I hang around. I hang out. I don't have to "make a career". For me, social connections are my top priority, dinner, theater, eating together with friends. In my practice in Bern I take forty-five minutes for lunch, just for lunch, nothing else, unlike my colleagues who go through clinic notes or catch up on professional journals while they eat. I also try to arrange Shiatsu exchanges with colleagues, but this doesn't happen often enough. I also forget work when I have a private life. Maybe just hanging around reflects the African side of me?
Madina Bokoum: Shiatsu Therapist, Counselor and Teacher, Zurich, Switzerland

The key sign of burnout as an actor is when I view my work as a job. I often feel this way during, say, the eighth performance in a week, on that wearisome Sunday night before the one precious day off. This is quickly rectified by making sure I re-connect with nature the next day. I try to keep burnout at bay by being quiet, reading mysteries, playing with our two adorable cats. But the primary restorer is being outside, walking briskly along the beach or up a mountain. I also try to maintain a regular practice of mindfulness meditation.... .
Megan Cole MA: Actor of Stage and TV and creator of workshops to teach physician/patient interaction skills to medical and nursing students. Nehalem, Oregon

I get energy from helping people feel better. However I do have to discharge, release, generate and re-integrate myself, and do this through dance and movement, forms such as Bonnie Bainbridge Cohen's Body-Mind Centering, Gabrielle Roth's 5 Rhythm Wave work, Contact Improv and Authentic Movement. Dance influences the way I work with people—especially the "Contact Improv"—a post modern dance form—because it requires you to listen, to be attentive to where the other person is, and to sense how things will move. I also do more ecstatic dance—I feel fields of energy, and I discharge my stagnant *Ki*. This generates and integrates balance—and emotions.

Jeffrey Dann PhD, LAc, AOBTA®-CI: Acupuncturist, Medical Anthropologist and Teacher, Boulder Colorado

Introspection. Yoga for clarity of thought. Swimming under water in silence. Solitude. Listening to waterfalls or the ocean and the sound of waves. Giggling with friends.

Debra Duncan Persinger PhD, DipTchg: Executive Director, Federation of State Massage Therapy Boards. Overland Park, Kansas

Burnout signs—tiredness in the afternoon, a tendency to want to isolate myself, stay at home or in bed reading crime stories and hating phone calls. I avoid this by taking breaks, a big midday break on a long day, for walking or swimming, and a three week break two times a year, at least, and a small break of ten days around Christmas. I've also taken more time for family and friends ever since we bought a house in France in 1997.

Anna Christa Endrich: Co-Director, *European Shiatsu Institute*, Heidelberg, Germany

I recognize burnout in myself when I don't diagnose (by seeing people as a great work of art), but when I grasp onto a symptom and treat that instead of the whole person. It's easy and you don't have to be present. You get tired when you check out during a session. You need to come back to your breath.

Barbra Esher LAc, Dipl Ac & ABT (NCCAOM) AOBTA®-CI, BFA: Acupuncturist, Shiatsu Teacher, former President and Director of Education, AOBTA®, Baltimore Maryland

I rejuvenate by following my passions, writing, classical music (especially Mozart), cycling, creating a magnificent garden, deep friendships, art museums, theater, books, community activism, and exploring my Celtic roots in Cornwall as often as I can. I well know the warning signs of burnout—over-giving and a lack of *Qi* and joy when I teach workshops or treat patients, lack of creative thought, and deep melancholy.

Pamela Ellen Ferguson Dipl ABT (NCCAOM), AOBTA®-CI, GSD, LMT: International Teacher of Shiatsu, and Author of eight books. Austin, Texas

I love teaching so much that the actual teaching doesn't burn me out. What does burn me out is the paperwork that goes with it like tests and evaluation reports.

Self-Care is very important. I prefer to receive Shiatsu when I get worked on but I need a skilled person to meet my needs, and one who can see me on a regular basis. If I can't find that in a Shiatsu practitioner, I will look for those qualities in a Bodyworker who practices another form of treatment that feels right for me. Currently I get Alexander Technique every week, massage every other week, chiropractic as needed. I do Pilates and Yoga every week. This isn't a luxury. It's a minimum of maintenance for someone my age (60) who still does 20 treatments per week. Also—I take a vacation!

Lindy Ferrigno Dipl ABT (NCCAOM) AOBTA®-CI, LMT: Shiatsu Therapist and Teacher, Charlottesville Virginia

I go to the woods. I get treated regularly. Really, the greatest healer is the wilderness. One of my teachers, J.R. Worsley, told me I would learn more from little children and nature, than from any Acupuncture book. But I think we need conferences for healing grief—and for healers' grief where we can just work on one another. We listen to suffering and misery all day and it's a big problem. I feel burnout and then someone calls and says their house is on fire and I think "your house fire is worse than mine" and I treat them. You end up frying yourself in the process.

David Ford LAc: Acupuncturist and creator of Taoist Wilderness based training in the Five Elements. Alaska, Oregon and New Zealand

I never take myself too seriously. Swimming helps. As does eating, drinking, sleeping, reading and any other—ing that you fancy. I just move on. Stop burning and compassioning.

Andrew Gamble LAc: Acupuncturist, Chinese Herbalist, and Co-Author of *Chinese Herbal Medicine: Materia Medica.* **Massachussetts**

I practice a tradition of yoga cultivated and disseminated by B.K.S. Iyengar. I eat nutritious food, drink a lot of water, and avoid alcohol. Participate in private psychotherapy. Take Chinese Herbs and nutritional supplements. Take Acupuncture every three weeks, and massage once a month. Do not own a TV. I know my limit on the number of patients I can treat in one week. I pace my day. I never work when I'm sick. When I sense I am at my limit in terms of giving out, I stop and rest from caring for others and care for myself.

Kathleen Golden LAc, MS: Acupuncturist and pioneer of outreach Acupuncture clinics for disaster zones. New York City

I have learned to be present and in the moment. This and regular meditation helps prevent burnout. Honestly burnout is not a problem for me like it was when I worked in hospitals. I am in control of my schedule now. I have the time to spend with a client, to build a rapport with them. I spend an hour with each client, and one and a half to two hours with new clients. The average MD has seven minutes with a client—how can you learn anything in that time? I'm concerned about Acupuncturists falling into the same sad situation. That sounds like a recipe for burnout.

Anne Gray BS, RT (T), LAc, MSOM: Acupuncturist, Teacher, Austin Texas, and former director, School of Radiation Therapy, Department of Radiation Oncology, Memorial Sloan—Kettering Cancer Center, New York City

For me, it is essential to keep myself nourished with my art, good food, plenty of rest, moderate exercise, plus regular treatments and Bodywork. When things are right in my world I can balance work and play. I enjoy my practice and I feel creative in my treatment style. When I'm overdoing it, the first thing to fall out of my schedule is painting. There doesn't seem to be time to take care of myself and I lose my playfulness. Painting is soul food, it lets me know where I am. It synchronizes me with the universe and the flow.

Karen Greathouse LAc, MSOM, BA (Fine Arts): Acupuncturist and Artist, Austin, Texas, and Mexico City

My warning sign is when I am just going through the motions. I have a couple of Acupuncture "formulas" that help just about anyone feel good in the moment, but basically do nothing for the duration. When I find myself doing that I need to take notice. Usually I need time for myself, whether meditative time, exercise, or physical work that is completely removed from the medicine. Consciousness of the burnout and moving in an opposite direction fixes it for me. Avoiding burnout is doing those curative things before the burnout begins.

Lesley Hamilton LAc, MSOM: Acupuncturist and Teacher, Austin, Texas

Avoid burnout by taking frequent breaks during the day, deep breathing (a lot!), getting away often (even if it's for a few minutes of meditation), maintaining a strong connection with the natural world, staying physically active, practicing Qigong, stretching every evening, eating well (with occasional splurges, including adult beverages), taking a few dietary supplements, learning new things every day, and sharing fun times with family and friends. Burnout warning signs, fatigue, irritability, aches and pains, tight muscles and joints, trouble sleeping, anxiety/depression and overeating.

Debra Howard Dipl ABT (NCCAOM) AOBTA®-CI, LMT: Teacher, and former President of AOBTA®, New Orleans, Louisiana

It's difficult for me to take care of my personal needs—I've always, since childhood, learned to see what others need, but never what I need. There are moments when I feel paralyzed inside. I'm learning ways of taking care of my "wood" energy by moving, doing Qigong, jogging, and having good structures in my everyday life. When I'm depressed I listen to good music (especially Andreas Scholl, Huelgas Ensemble, Handel). My little daughter Karoline also helps me to find distance from work and worries.

Beate Johl, Physical Therapist, Shiatsu Teacher, and Translator, Berlin, Germany

Don't work too long with a patient. Get to know how long is too long for you. Get out of your treatment room into nature and let the elements blow through you. Clear your room after each treatment. Wash your hands and arms in cold running water. Take regular breaks. Be with your client during the treatment but not afterwards. Keep your distance.

John McKeever: Director, *Shiatsu School Belfast*, Northern Ireland

My Shiatsu attitude is: not doing, not working. Just being present, observant, accompanying, not interfering. Yes, this sounds very much like a well known Zen paradox—plain philosophy—and I must admit, that I managed to put this into practice only after a long practical experience of Shiatsu work (since 1981). It doesn't automatically work always, as I am still developing. Anyway, this attitude gives me space to be aware of myself while "working." It acknowledges that in Shiatsu there are always two, enclosing the wellbeing of the receiver and giver alike at the same time.

Klaus Metzner: Director, *European Shiatsu Institute*, Munich, Germany

If you are giving, giving, giving all the time and not receiving, your psyche knows this and it will let you know about the imbalance somehow. Health is about *Qi* and *Qi* exchange. I know my own warning signs of burnout. I get pushy with my patients. I want them to get better. I push them and then feel tired at the end of the day. That's usually a sign I need to take care of myself more. I took a sabbatical after twenty two years of practice and twenty seven years as a psychotherapist. Right now I'm finding teaching more rewarding—I'm affecting people that can affect people. I do Qigong, get Bodywork, travel. I go to Italy where my ancestors are from, for renewal, to enjoy life. I think more about that as I grow older. That whole stream of ancestral energy—what does it offer me? How do I best embody what I have to offer?

Lorena Monda LAc, OMD, MS: Acupuncturist, Psychotherapist and Teacher, Albuquerque, New Mexico

I avoid burnout by varying my activities. I write, teach, and study new methodologies. This keeps me inspired and on top of the game while creating enough variation to keep up the good work. During the day it is important to be reflective and mindful of disconnecting between patients. Washing the hands is a perfect moment for this practice.

William Morris DAOM, LAc: President *Academy of Oriental Medicine at Austin,* Texas

If I fail to tell my family and friends that I have the best job in the world I know I need to take some time off. I know that I am at my healing best when I am healthy. I try to be proactive in this by taking off on Friday afternoons at 1 pm. This has worked well to give me time to get some kind of Bodywork on a weekly basis including Acupuncture, Massage, Chiropractic or Cranial Sacral Therapy to prevent burnout. That's my time for me.

Karen Nunley LAc, MSOM: Acupuncturist and Teacher, Austin, Texas

I take time out regularly, do a lot of sports, especially competition sport, laugh and love, have fun and be lazy.

Roberto Preinreich, Director, *European Shiatsu Institute*, Vienna, Austria

I do Qigong every day. When I'm tired I use Qigong to help relax my mind and to see things clearly.

Yuxia Qiu LAc, MD (China): Acupuncturist, Calligrapher, Teacher of Acupuncture Techniques, Nutrition, Qigong and Tai Chi, *Academy of Oriental Medicine at Austin,* Texas

I try to do what I *love* to do. I exercise and meditate daily. I respect and accept any turbulence, physical as well as psychological in my life, as a sign that I am growing, knowing this takes time and patience. I accept that I am getting older and have to cut down a bit.

Wilfried Rappenecker Dr. Med: Shiatsu Teacher, Physician, and owner of *Shiatsu Schule Hamburg*, Germany

By getting enough sleep. By regular exercise like practicing Yoga, and by receiving regular Shiatsu. By finding and living my own life rhythm.

Bernhard Ruhla: Physical Therapist, Shiatsu and Yoga Teacher, Dresden, Germany

Burnout for me is an emotional state when I don't want to connect, and avoid spending time on any given task. My fuse is short. My outlook becomes gray. I feel flat, dry. When I sense these warning signs, I pace myself, give myself time-outs. I nourish myself by connecting to helpful friends, to beauty, to music (especially Beethoven's Fifth Symphony) to art—especially the Impressionists—and Monet's paintings of Haystacks and Water Lilies.

Jan Ste Germaine LAc, AOBTA®-CI: Acupuncturist and Shiatsu Teacher. Former vice president AOBTA®. Kansas City, Missouri

Follow the three aspects of mind, breath and good posture. To avoid burnout you must also train high *Ki* energy through exercise. It's something very basic.

Tetsuro Saito BSc, RMT, CST: known as the "Father of Shiatsu" in Toronto, Canada

Avoid burnout by first and foremost taking care of yourself. Receive wellness treatments from a variety of practitioners regularly. Laugh every day! Remind yourself of the magnificence of the human body. Spend at least 20 minutes outdoors everyday. Meet with colleagues on a regular basis. Keep balance in your personal and professional life. Be sure to have some friends that are not directly connected to your work. Be active in your community. Pace yourself well, eat healthy foods, exercise, and meditate.

Cherie Sohnen-Moe BA: Teacher and co-author *"The Ethics of Touch"*. Tucson, Arizona

I go to spas, to saunas and warm swimming pools—that's very important for me to rejuvenate. Also I spend a lot of time in the bathtub, and time in bed alone, being quiet, no telephone, no noise, just being. And it's wonderful to escape to my house in Spain, to be in the garden....

Edith Storch Shiatsu Instructor and school owner, *Shiatsu Zentrum Edith Storch*, Berlin, Germany

I heal my spirit with a practice of gratitude for all that I have. I heal my body with continued enjoyment of the physical world, with attention to enjoyment of exercise, food and sleep. I heal my mind with the right "livelihood" which continues to engage my interest and curiosity. I get tired and so I'll rest. I get overwhelmed and I'll eliminate something which feels pressing. I get stressed and I'll look to ease my burden. Burnout is easily avoided by following the medicine we practice.
Maryanne Travaglione LAc: Acupuncturist and Teacher, Brooklyn, New York

Don't identify with your job too much. Avoid the *Helfer-Syndrom*, the tendency to want to save the world. Such "crusaders" rely too much on their jobs for emotional confirmation—and that's very dangerous! I'm not only a practitioner and teacher, but a husband, father, and friend. Do things just for your own life "leave your job" completely from time to time. I do this by walking my horse (together with a friend if possible) through the forests for hours or a day or longer. Take a Buddhist approach. Look at the world with a cheerful calmness. Sometimes I laugh at myself, my life and my ideas, to balance the seriousness and the problems confronting me.
Eduard Tripp DPhil: Shiatsu Teacher, Psychotherapist, Editor, Vienna, Austria

As a therapist you must be "kind" to yourself. Some therapists feel they must be on call all the time for their clients. You need to recognize the limits of your abilities. Too many of us feel we have not "done enough" for a client. Develop interests apart from your practice. Spending time on other activities allows you to get perspective on your work, and you return to it and your patients with a refreshed mind. I have a great interest in nature and get out as much as possible to study butterflies, dragonflies, plants and birds. Time away from my practice is invaluable and enhances my overall well-being.
Nancy van der Poorten BSc, CST: Vice Principal Emerita, *Shiatsu School of Canada,* and currently studying butterfly ecology in Sri Lanka

I would say exercise daily. Take personal space as much as you can. Take vacations without computers and cell phones. Take time away, come back refreshed. Have a good staff. Cultivate patients who understand you are not always there.
Stuart Watts LAc, AOBTA®-CI, and creator of schools of Asian Medicine, Austin, Texas

Good planning, freetime, vacations. Don't feel you have to save the world. Keep a healthy distance from your patients, while still being empathetic. Be compassionate but don't suffer with them. Have fun in the evenings, go jogging. Let go of overload. Do whatever you can to relax.

Carien Wijnen Dr Med: Dutch born physician, choir teacher and song writer, Berlin Germany

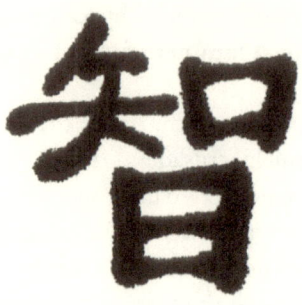

WISDOM—calligraphy by Yuxia Qiu, LAc

B: THE WORKPLACE

Professors of Education at New York University never lectured on how to handle flying-sandwich situations.—Frank McCourt. *Teacher Man (1)*

Thus while one may be horrified by the ravages of developmental disorder or disease, one may sometimes see them as creative, too—for if they destroy particular paths, particular ways of doing things, they may force the nervous system into making other paths and ways, force on it unexpected growth and evolution.—Oliver Sacks. *An Anthropologist on Mars (2)*

KINDNESS—calligraphy by Yuxia Qiu, LAc

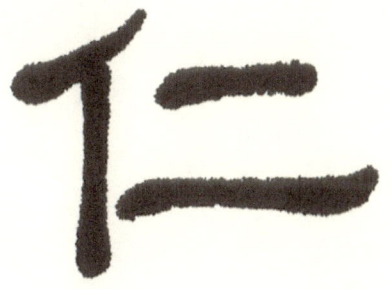

10

Creating a Shiatsu School in Berlin

EDITH STORCH: Certified Shiatsu Teacher (*Shiatsu Lehrerin—German Shiatsu Society)*, Certified Health Practitioner, *(Heilpraktikerin) Founder and Director, Shiatsu Zentrum Edith Storch, Berlin. Edith trained as a teacher for social work before starting her Shiatsu education in England in 1980, and completed her training through the Shiatsu Schule Berlin Hamburg in the mid 1980s. She created the first Shiatsu school for women in Germany.*

Q: What is your vision for the future growth of Shiatsu in Germany?

ES: When I started teaching in 1986, a regulated curriculum did not exist in Germany! My biggest wish was to develop new teaching content in the classes I was offering. We all started with the basics like meridians and Five Elements. At that time the training took about a year and a half. I found it challenging to expand that basic training and to offer new directions, for example, what is the best way to teach diagnosis, or, what is the most meaningful way to teach the changing phases of the Five Elements, and how do you spark a student's ability to be perceptive? Also, how can we integrate the challenges posed by everyday life for students and for practitioners, and how do we deal with diseases like AIDS for example?

Q: What made you decide to create the first Shiatsu School for Women?

ES: From the beginning I had a great interest in teaching women because the field of Bodywork offers a special learning atmosphere. Additionally, at that time, and still today, the theme of women's health is marginalized. In my experience, subjects like sexual abuse and child abuse and women's health themes are discussed more openly and in greater depth in a group of women only. Also, during my training, they would teach us to work right through the breast area for Stomach and other meridians for example and that made many of us uncomfortable, so we changed that aspect of the training. It was also very important for me to change the *language* of the training, not only to honor the feminine ending in words (in German) where previously only masculine terminology and endings were used. And to strip all violent language from the training, for example, the common use of the term *opfer* ("victim") for the student who volunteers to be the model in a demonstration. We also use charts and Acupuncture dolls showing the meridians on women and this is very unusual. Most charts show only the male outline even though most of the students are women.

Q: And yet among other innovations your Zentrum was the first in Germany to offer a weekend workshop on Men's Health!

ES: Yes and the students loved it!

Q: What are the other reasons why students choose your Zentrum?

ES: Sure enough the position of the Zentrum in Berlin-Kreuzberg attracts women from east and west, and also, the local Turkish women who don't join mixed classes. Kreuzberg also attracts a lot of alternative and politically conscious people who live and work there, and show a growing interest in alternative medicine. Our different teachers also influence the way the Zentrum is seen from the outside. Our teachers include mothers, single women, gay, straight, physiotherapists, and women from other branches of the health profession. Their ages range from 35–63. So the students are as diverse as the teachers, ranging in age from 19–65 an eclectic mix of women, single, divorced, physiotherapists, nurses, medical doctors, librarians, historians, Egyptologists, journalists, social workers, and also the unemployed and those seeking a second career. Educating this colorful mix of people is very typical of us and we love doing it!

Q: What is your vision for Shiatsu training in the future?

ES: For me the biggest question is how to make Shiatsu more mainstream. I integrate meditation, Feng Shui, Qigong and Nutrition into our Shiatsu training. I also include Shiatsu training on the table instead of the floor, and the students appreciate this option! I also teach NLP (Neuro Linguistic Programming) to help students develop their Q&A skills for clinical practice, and to be able to read a patient's body language, how patients react to certain questions and how they move their eyes and so on. And I teach Emotional Freedom techniques, where we *tap tap tap* an Acupuncture point to access psychological problems, and teach students how to be aware of changes in meridian patterns and emotional patterns during a session. My personal emphasis is on the connection between the psyche and Shiatsu. Our supervised praktikum is very important. But equally important is the opportunity for graduates to be supervised again and again at the Zentrum according to the guidelines of the Shiatsu Society of Germany. (GSD—*Gesellschaft fur Shiatsu Deutschland*).

Q: Do you see a change in the role of the German Shiatsu Society (GSD)?

ES: The GSD consolidated the strength of Shiatsu Teachers and assured professional standards of training. In the future I see the GSD becoming even more forceful in the professional political sector throughout Germany.

Q: And finally—how do you teach students to be aware of the warning signs of burnout?

ES: We first discuss this in class in terms of the number of treatments to give in a day. This varies from student to student. Some can do six a day, some less, and I advise them to find a balance that works for them. I tell them I used to treat six patients a day, three days a week, but don't work like that now I own a school!

I also tell them it's important for them to ask themselves how they feel. How is their energy? And if they work long hours, do they have a partner at home to do the housework, shopping and cooking? And I tell them to be aware of the early signs of burnout. To ask themselves—do I have fun with my work? Do I like my work? And to keep track of their health. Then I advise them to get treatments, being touched is very important.

11

Creating a Shiatsu School in Hamburg

WILFRIED RAPPENECKER Dr Med. Certified Shiatsu Teacher (*Shiatsule-hrer* German Shiatsu Society), *Acupuncturist, founder and director, Shiatsu Schule Hamburg, and program director of the International School of Shiatsu, Kiental Switzerland, where he initiated the European Shiatsu Congress in 2004 and 2007. Wilfried completed his medical studies in Germany and his Shiatsu studies through the Ohashi Institute New York City and with Saul Goodman in Kiental, Switzerland. He co-created two of Germany's earliest Shiatsu schools (in Hamburg and Berlin), and is the author of several major textbooks in the German language, including "Yu Sen", (1) "Funf Elemente und 12 Meridiane"(2) and "Atlas Shiatsu-Die Meridiane des Zen-Shiatsu" (3).*

Q: What inspired you to expand your MD training to include Acupuncture and Shiatsu?

WR: Well, to be honest: I believed that this was the best thing I could do to support my spiritual path. Although at that time in 1986 I would not have been able to define what a spiritual path was! It was just a very strong feeling. I did not think at that time that Shiatsu was more effective than modern scientific medicine, nor do I think that now. However, I discovered that Shiatsu has a lot more to offer than I thought in 1981. Shiatsu is a complete therapeutic discipline by itself. Studying Acupuncture was important for me to broaden my understanding about TCM and Shiatsu. I practiced it for a while. However, I hardly practice Acupuncture nowadays. I almost totally gave it up (as I gave up craniosacral work) because Shiatsu offers all the tools I need for my work.

Q: *You co-created two of the major Shiatsu schools in Germany. What new approaches/methods/topics did you introduce to the training in areas you felt were lacking in your own training?*

WR: OK, Shiatsu training today is entirely different from the training I received in the early 1980s. The most important aspects of our training right now that weren't included in my training in the early or late 1980s include: Five Element theory and practice in detail, anatomy and physiology, counseling skills, how to give advice to a client, transference and countertransference issues, energetic perceptions, Meridian-Free Shiatsu, Specialized Shiatsu for specific complaints, Shiatsu for clients with psychological problems, and how to open a practice. There is still quite a long way to go however. Personally I have developed a whole new understanding of Shiatsu. I do not see meridian work as the core of Shiatsu anymore.

As a tool in class I introduce something I call a "guided treatment"—guided by me, but involving five students. They decide which one of them should receive the treatment. Then the other four interview him/her, and one of them will perform the *Hara* or Back diagnosis, and they all discuss a treatment procedure. Then each one works on the receiver in sequences of about ten minutes. I share my observations, and ask them about the next steps, but in the end I decide on the best step and explain why. I may also lead their hands if they have difficulties finding the right depth, or the right angle. These treatments are quite intensive. Students learn about the flow of the treatment. They learn about the meaning of a clear topic and focus and how to understand the receiver's reactions. I also ask the students what they perceive at specific moments during the course of the treatment.

Q: *Can you explain Meridian-Free Shiatsu?*

WR: I perceive the body of my client as a space that—as any energy field—is structured into fields/areas of different qualities. I compare this view of the whole person with whatever the client tells me about his/her complaint. Then I decide which area of the body should get my first priority during the treatment. I perceive the pattern of a focus area. When it changes during a treatment I see this as a sign that my work is effective. I find this interesting and rewarding. We still teach meridians, but we consider them just one important tool in Shiatsu besides others. Meridian-Free energetic orientation in the body becomes the core of Shiatsu. On the other hand meridian work has been further developed. We distinguish between energetic organs and meridians. We also work with the psychological aspect of an organ by staying in contact with a client's ability to focus on the central function of an organ and to perceive the changes in it while we work along a corresponding meridian.

Q: *Do you personally teach your students the necessary counseling skills in your school?*

WR: Yes I do, in connection with the diagnostic process. In the past we also tried inviting psychologists (who were not Shiatsu practitioners). But this didn't work. There was either too much misunderstanding, or the person could not relate to Shiatsu.

Q: *Can you describe the sort of cases you share with your students where you combine your western medical knowledge with your Shiatsu diagnoses and treatments?*

WR: Let's take the case of lower back pain. Here modern medicine follows quite a mechanical route (slipped disc, protrusion or prolapse, etc.). The energetic view however, makes a lot more sense and offers more possibilities in treatment. The Shiatsu view also offers a model of understanding as to why so many extremely painful conditions show no—or only slightly—altered discs. Whereas frequently, slipped discs can be found in patients experiencing no pain. In the case of a stiff neck, the energetic situation, including psychological issues, are usually much more important than the model of the trapped nerve.

Other cases I teach in class involve psychological issues such as depression and states of anxiety. Here I find that the energetic model often offers a solution that is much more real than the standard understanding of looking for the causes of what happened in the past. However we do discuss such aspects as the students are very interested. In my clinical experience, therapeutic Shiatsu works best on—muscular-skeletal problems you meet in physiotherapy such as lower back pain, knee problems, pain therapy, menstrual problems, but also headaches and insomnia, postoperative rehabilitation, functional disorders of internal organ systems and on clients with psychological problems of various kinds including Post Traumatic Stress Disorder, and those who need a new orientation through a difficult time in life.

Q: *How do you teach your students to recognize problems that are beyond the scope of practice of Shiatsu, and need to be referred to an MD?*

WR: This is taught by one of our teachers for anatomy, physiology and pathology. Principally it is about teaching students to recognize the symptoms of serious and life threatening illness like acute abdominal problems, heart attack or failure, emboli of the lungs, stroke, thrombosis etc.

Q: *You use the term "therapeutic Shiatsu" a lot. Do you mean advanced (medical) use of Shiatsu to diagnose and treat a specific health problem, compared with, say, just a fitness center—or—spa Shiatsu?*

WR: Yes that's exactly what I mean, because I find there is a widespread misunderstanding about the role Shiatsu can play, and some believe that clients with more specific illnesses should be referred to some "real" therapy. There have been many discussions in the German Shiatsu Society (GSD) about this, when, for political reasons, the GSD suggested dropping the term "therapeutic" in connection with Shiatsu, and for that reason many practitioners no longer felt at home in the GSD. I believe in the therapeutic potential which, to my understanding, is the same as that of psychotherapy, physiotherapy or other forms of Bodywork like craniosacral work.

Q: *You describe German society as among the most conservative, especially re the wider integration of Shiatsu in hospitals and clinics. And yet many Shiatsu students in Germany are physiotherapists who take the work into hospitals and clinics.*

WR: But very few of them practice Shiatsu openly, and Health Insurance does not reimburse them for Shiatsu. On the other hand, physiotherapists practicing Shiatsu in private practice or hospitals provide a way for the medical establishment to discover the therapeutic potential of Shiatsu. We've invited Shiatsu Practitioners with hospital experience in the USA to give a speech at our university hospital. I believed that if someone comes with the recommendation of a heart surgeon, then other doctors will be more open to what he has to share. It looks like I'm right!

12

Creating Schools of Acupuncture in the USA

STUART WATTS, LAc, OMD, AOBTA®-CI *has created several leading schools of Acupuncture in the USA, and serves on a number of national boards including the National Qigong Association (NQA), and the American Organization for Bodywork Therapies of Asia, AOBTA®. During 2006 he created the American Association for Teachers of Acupuncture and Oriental Medicine (AATAOM) and the Foundation for the Advancement of Asian Medicine to provide scholarships to students, and to document the history of Asian Medicine in the West.*

Q: *You are widely known in the USA for creating schools in New Mexico and Texas. Can you summarize your pioneering evolution through Chinese Medicine?*

SW: I started studying Chinese Medicine around 1972 when there was very little information available in the United States and only a handful of instructors. By the end of 1976 I was fortunate enough to have studied with most of them. In 1977 The New England School of Acupuncture opened in Boston, Massachusetts and I completed their one-year program before continuing my studies in England (where I was born).

Then I moved to Canada to open up an Asian Bodywork program with three teachers of Herbology and martial arts. Once this was up and going, I traveled to Santa Fe to teach various classes at the Santa Fe College of Natural Medicine and to start a program in Acupuncture in 1980. At that time it was only the fourth or fifth program in the United States. It was a two-year, 1,800 hour program and cost $800 a year. A few years later I co-created the not-for-profit Institute of Traditional Medicine with programs in Naturopathic Medicine, Western Herbology, Nutrition, Massage, and Ayurvedic Medicine and of course Chinese Medicine. Eventually the Chinese Medicine part siphoned off to became the International Institute of Chinese Medicine.

Later I created the Southwest Acupuncture College. SWAC continues to this day with locations in Santa Fe and Albuquerque, New Mexico and Boulder, Colorado. I then traveled the world before moving to Austin Texas to open a clinic. By then, in 1993, Chinese Medicine was more evolved. There were about 25 schools in the country (today there are about 55). I started the Academy of Oriental Medicine at the local Austin community's request. It grew from under 20 students to over 300 today. I sold it in 2000 when it offered a comprehensive 3,200 hour program spread over four years. Considered one of the top three schools in the USA, AOMA reflected my own growth as a practitioner and educator. I created a fully integrated program that included Chinese Herbology, Tai Chi, Qigong, Asian Bodywork Therapy (Shiatsu, and Tuina) and good counseling skills. The initial program was about 2,800 hours when most schools were about 1,800.

My main goal in developing schools was to provide outstanding education for students and outstanding practitioners for the community. I have lived up to that dream.

Q: *What innovations did you introduce in your schools?*

SW: Chinese Medicine is more than just about sticking in needles. When I first attended a school that was about all there was, and limited reference material. I introduced both nutrition and Bodywork (Shiatsu and Tuina) to the Acupuncture program as being an essential part of the training. Bodywork was of paramount importance—how can you stick needles into a patient without an accomplished touch? Everyone needs and loves to be touched. This was very unique at the time, though some textbooks existed in Shiatsu and Acupressure. There were very few books on Acupuncture at that time, and most of the material was photocopied from various sources. Today, textbooks on Acupuncture and related subjects are in abundance compared with the paucity of material in those early days of Chinese Medical education in the USA.

I also introduced extensive herbal training into the curriculum right from the beginning. It was mostly Western Herbal Medicine but soon included Chinese Herbal Medicine. The program was also an expression of compassion, communication, and community. We weren't a disassociated group of individuals. We shared a lot in those days. We introduced training in practitioner/patient interaction skills, teaching students how to *listen*.

What we were really studying was art and history. We inspired students to explore and experiment with Chinese Medicine, and to continue studying other forms of medicine. I realized that to be really great, one also needed to accomplish internal arts such as Qigong and meditation. How could one practice medicine without some kind of inner understanding? The training in any Acupuncture school of mine was not going to be one of just education, but of self-education. I wanted to push my students to the point where they changed as people. I also wanted a very strong clinical component. We did that and still maintain standards that are generally higher or equal to the highest requirements in clinical training in the United States (usually New Mexico or Hawaii).

We were also able to acquire an amazing group of teachers from China here in Austin that made AOMA a great gathering of scholars who could actually teach many aspects of the medicine that were unknown to us in the early 70's and 80's.

Q: How has the regulation/licensing of Acupuncture evolved in the last few decades?

SW: In the 1980s during the time of the Santa Fe schools, the political situation did not encourage Chinese Medicine. It was illegal in most states including New Mexico. So we had to prompt change. This inspired a group of us to become politicized. We were able to change the law in New Mexico in 1982 to allow licensing. We also helped form national organizations, AAAOM, NCCAOM, CCAOM, and ACAOM (though some acronyms have changed from their original names). It was very inspiring to develop these organizations with our graduates, and to get students involved in the politics of Acupuncture when they moved to other states to practice.

The medicine has become more standardized, more mainstream. The educational material has become more (though not totally) standardized.

We now have accreditation boards to oversee schools. There are testing agencies that examine the graduates of institutions. There are professional state boards. Thirty six states now have licensing laws. Programs in education have become more standardized. This is of course a big difference from the days when schools didn't have to live up to any standard. Today the top schools offer Master's and some offer Doctoral degrees often sought by graduates in a range of other professions (medical, the arts, engineering, computer sciences, management etc) who seek second or third careers. There are even incentives for those switching from military careers into the healing profession.

These days most students have to study Chinese Herbology and extended hours in Western Medicine, and complete a higher number of clinical hours than was required years ago.

In addition, there are now certification requirements for Asian Bodywork Therapists which have raised the standards in the country.

Q: *Did you always aim to strike a balance in your schools between Western instructors and Chinese instructors?*

SW: I believe that an institution of Chinese Medicine in the West needs a combination of teachers from both cultures. I find that the best balance is a 50–50 split. I also believe that there is a lot of potential growth among teachers that are Westerners and have developed the medicine to fit the needs of Western students and patients.

The Chinese bring to the classroom the experience of using the medicine in a setting where the patient can visit on a regular basis without a major cost (though currently things are becoming more privatized). The practitioner gets to see what really works and what does not. They also get to work in collaboration with other practitioners in an integrated hospital setting.

In addition, studying Chinese Medicine in China is really different. They have thousands of years of experience and the textbooks are in their native language. This allows for a fuller understanding of the medicine and for greater depth of discussion. Western teachers bring an understanding of the culture in which their students and patients live. Social, financial and emotional realities in the west are very different from China. The combination of teachers really makes for the best education. It also allows for the growth of Chinese Medicine here in the West to adapt to the Western mind set.

Q: *What advice do you give new instructors from China to help them adapt to teaching in America?*

SW: It is always hard to change cultural settings with understanding. American students are very different from Chinese students, so it's important for new instructors from China to observe classes taught by Chinese colleagues who have been in America for sometime, and to observe Western instructors as well. Unfortunately most schools would not facilitate this, as they need to pay the teacher who just arrived from China who is probably supporting his/her family.

Q: *If you created an Acupuncture school today, how different would it be from your other schools?*

SW: Ideally I would develop an internship program. I believe that this what current programs in Chinese Medicine lack. I would add another year or eight months to the program where the graduate could be monitored or mentored by a practitioner. The biggest problem today is the graduate leaving school and lacking confidence. I just think graduates could all use a bit more time. I also believe that adding an internship program should be required for a Doctoral program.

Q: *Would you encourage the expansion of internships, in hospitals, clinics, etc?*

SW: If Chinese Medicine is going to survive in the USA, it has to be integrated into the health system to include clinics, public health and hospitals. This is happening slowly. Every year there are more and more practitioners practicing in typically Western settings. Schools are having associations with local communities and community clinics. If we were to integrate Chinese Medicine into national legislation such as Medicare then the general approval by traditional Western health settings and insurance companies would increase dramatically, but more for Acupuncture than for Chinese Herbal medicine.

With today's prices of studying Chinese Medicine in the USA, there has to be a wider way for graduates to make a decent living. The typical student coming out of Chinese Medical school is in debt to the Federal Student Loan program from $60,000—$80,000 dollars or more. This is too much of a burden on the graduate if the medicine is not accepted by the mainstream. They simply won't be able to make a living, or will combine a practice with a prior profession, like teaching or computer science.

Q: You are famous for highlighting Asian Bodywork Therapy in your schools, more than most schools, some of which have barely any ABT training at all. Do any of your colleagues in other schools ever challenge/question your emphasis on ABT?

SW: I'm always being challenged by others in my profession for the work that I do in Asian Bodywork. I'm kind of amazed. Most of this comes from those who are not really practitioners but educators and trying to get graduates out of school as fast as they can, without really understanding the fullness of the medicine. Asian Bodywork is the basis and foundation of the medicine. You must be able to touch the patient to do Acupuncture. You have to touch the patient to "know" the patient.

It is not only important for a practitioner to work on other people but also themselves. Like Tai Chi or Qigong they need to feel the *Qi* in themselves—where it moves and where it is blocked. By working on themselves, they see the benefits of Bodywork on a very practical and personal level. This translates into being able to touch the patient and feel energy blocks. This is a major part of diagnosis and treatment. It is said that touch diagnosis is 90% accurate. Touch is a form of communication. Communication is a major part of healing.

To learn to do professional Asian Bodywork Therapy on a patient takes time in theory and in practice. Most schools are in a hurry with their students to get them to learn theory, Acupuncture, Herbs, Western medical principles and don't want to take the time necessary in the schooling to explore Bodywork. It's so practical to learn Asian Bodywork while learning basic theory in general Chinese Medical education, because it gives students so much applied experience. The student can complete this part of their education in the first or second year of training, and can start an ABT practice while they complete their Acupuncture and Herbal training over the next three years. This helps develop invaluable clinical skills, and can help offset the cost of student loans. Patients love Bodywork, usually even more than needling.

Sadly however, Asian Bodywork is really not a big part of the accreditation process or the standard curriculum required of schools, so it tends to be avoided by many schools. It should be taught by all schools.

Q: What new waves are you aiming to make through your newest innovations, your foundation, and a very different organization for instructors?

SW: Probably the most important organization that I have created recently is the American Association for Teachers of Acupuncture and Oriental Medicine (AATAOM). This organization creates a forum for teachers of all aspects of Asian Medicine to communicate with each other. It is specifically designed to improve a teacher's ability to teach. Many teachers of Asian Medicine are either Chinese in origin or clinical people who have been asked to teach a class. To be a teacher is to be a professional teacher. AATAOM will provide experienced teachers ways in which they can improve their skills.

The other organization that I have created is the Foundation for the Advancement of Asian Medicine, a not-for-profit 501(c)(3) organization designed to do two things: to provide scholarships for students at approved schools, and to inspire tax-deductible donations. The Foundation is also documenting the history of Chinese Medicine in the USA, including filming the founders of the Medicine in modern history.

13

From Shiatsu in Canada to Butterflies in Sri Lanka

NANCY VAN DER POORTEN, BS (Botany), CST, *Member, Shiatsu Therapy Association of Ontario (STAO), and Vice-Principal Emerita of the Shiatsu School of Canada. Nancy and her husband Michael are currently on sabbatical in Sri Lanka, studying life cycles of butterflies and dragonflies, and promoting conservation and butterfly gardens. She was a major contributor to the North American Journal of Oriental Medicine (NAJOM), and a former Vice-President of the Shiatsu Therapy Association of Ontario (STAO)*

Q: *In your years at the helm of one of Canada's leading Shiatsu schools, what innovations in training did you introduce?*

NvdP: Because the school was regulated by the provincial government, we had to follow a set curriculum and set hours within which we had some leeway. There was one course, *Auxiliary Modalities,* in which we could teach whatever we wanted and we used that to teach *Sotai* (corrective exercise), Moxibustion, Kinesiology, Chinese Herbs, Acupuncture (especially the Japanese style), Tuina etc. We felt this exposed students to the wider world of Asian Medicine as well as to some practical work with the body. We also arranged for the students to view cadavers at the chiropractic college—an optional visit but everyone went and learned a lot.

We also had the students do a series of treatments on one person—we realized that many students did not have the opportunity to treat an individual on an ongoing basis in a supervised setting so that they didn't see what a series of eight or ten weekly treatments could do. The student would either arrange to bring in someone from outside or could work with a fellow student. This was a most valuable exercise—it allowed the student to have the opportunity to treat the same person week after week, to see their concerns and how the treatment was affecting them. If the student was the one receiving treatments, it also allowed them to experience the benefits of treatment and to analyze their own responses. The instructor led a guided discussion after each session in which students were required to report on what they had done and the results and difficulties. At the end of the series of sessions, they had to submit a full report.

We also required the students to keep complete records of all the treatments done at the school. In-class treatments required more extensive notations while in-clinic treatments required a bit less. The students had to identify the chief complaint, results of the last treatment, goal for this treatment, and MITA—Most Important Treatment Areas. We based the record-keeping on the SOAP protocol—Subjective, Objective, Assessment and Plan—which we studied formally. We focused on written notes as well as graphical representations.

Q: Did you also organize off-site clinics?

NvdP: We also did many 'shows' with the students—setting up a booth and offering Shiatsu treatments. This allowed the students to have the opportunity to meet the general public, to learn how to explain Shiatsu to them, and to practice mini-sessions of 10–15 minutes. The students always enjoyed this activity and were highly energized and motivated by it.

We had a special Senior's Day when we offered free treatments to senior citizens. This gave the students the opportunity to work on a specific clientele and offered something back to the community.

At one time, we offered free mini-treatments to women at a local drop-in centre, and also required the students to arrange, organize and do a presentation in the community to a group of their choosing. This was a very valuable training for them. Unfortunately we had to drop offsite clinics because of the complicated liability insurance issues for the school in case of injury.

One thing that we were not allowed to do by the provincial authorities that I think is extraordinarily valuable was to have the students do practical internships at an outside clinic, or even at the school clinic. I believe that students must get experience of the business side of running a clinic as well as giving treatments.

Answering the phone, making appointments, cleaning the rooms, explaining things to the clients etc. are all part of one's daily life as a Shiatsu Therapist and I would have liked to have been able to require students to get this training either outside or in the school clinic. The authorities didn't allow this as they viewed it as us requiring the students to work or as fobbing off teaching hours. I would love to see the students being able to do more in the community and in hospital settings but the legal and insurance ramifications make it difficult to arrange.

Q: How do Shiatsu students get registered in Ontario?

NvdP: Students require 2,200 hours to join the Shiatsu Therapy Association of Ontario as a Certified Shiatsu Therapist (CST). There is no other 'registration' of Shiatsu Therapists except for some local government regulations. For example, the City of Toronto requires that a Shiatsu Therapist be licensed as a Holistic Practitioner. In order to get this license, you need to be a CST.

Training and the regulations concerning who can practice Shiatsu Therapy differ from province to province. There are no federal guidelines. In most provinces, anybody can practice Shiatsu Therapy though there may be restrictions on what titles they can use. The 2,200-hour training in Ontario is the highest in the country but there are also many schools in Ontario, and the other provinces, that offer anything from 100 to 1,100 hours.

Q: What were your major legislative achievements and what campaigns would you like your graduates to carry in your absence?

NvdP: Shiatsu Therapists have always been free to practice in the province of Ontario; however, we did fail to win status as a regulated health profession despite mighty efforts over the years. In local politics, Shiatsu Therapists managed to get their professional standing recognized by the city of Toronto when they brought in a Licensed Holistic Practitioner bylaw but have had to keep the pressure up to maintain this recognition. Graduates must keep an eye on these issues and continue to promote their best interests (which by definition must include the best interests of the clients as well).

The biggest challenge that I see is to get recognition from the insurance industry. Many people get coverage for treatments through their Extended Health

Care plans. This coverage often includes treatments done by an RMT, Registered Massage Therapist, even if they do Shiatsu Therapy for which they have had no training! For many years, we have been trying to get the CST (Certified Shiatsu Therapist) designation of the Shiatsu Therapy Association of Ontario recognized as the standard for Shiatsu Therapy. I think that this is the single most important thing that can now be done.

Q: You also wrote copious articles for the Shiatsu Society Journal and the North American Journal of Oriental Medicine. Are we doing enough for the modern evolution of Shiatsu to document case studies, new material & discoveries in our work with cancer, AIDS, PTSD, depression and so on for the next generation of students?

NvdP: Definitely not! I feel that Shiatsu Therapy will never move forward until we put ourselves on a more professional footing by doing research (which includes but is not confined to documenting case histories) and preparing material related to standards of practice, treatment guidelines, ethical issues etc. Until this is done, Shiatsu Therapy will retain a reputation as being a 'nice' but 'home-remedy' treatment. I would love to see Shiatsu Therapy be seriously respected as a primary treatment method (for the appropriate conditions of course) and as a very useful supportive treatment method. But this will not happen until there are written guidelines in place and until therapists themselves can elucidate their treatment goals and plans, diagnosis and results in a coherent and standard way.

Q: Has your current involvement in butterfly farms/Ecology made you wonder if the ideal future training in Shiatsu (or any form of Asian Medicine) should include training in—or a conscious observation of—our healing role in Ecology?

NvdP: I believe that a sensitive understanding of humans as an integral part of nature is helpful for all human beings, those doing the healing work, as well as those needing to be healed. But I find that the majority of people have no real interest and this is difficult to instill. Many children seem to have an intrinsic interest in nature that somehow gets lost for some as they get older.

14

Outreach Clinics for Disaster Areas and City Hospitals

KATHLEEN GOLDEN, LAc, MS *is a faculty member at Tri-State College of Acupuncture (TCSA) New York, specializing in women's health, public health and the application of essential oils in an Acupuncture practice. Apart from her private practice, she holds a clinical position at Village Care New York, an AIDS Day treatment program, where she won an Excellence in Service Award in 2007 for ten years of care. Kathleen served as President of the Acupuncture Society of New York for five years and was given the "Acupuncturist of the Year" award by the American Association of Oriental Medicine in 2000. She is a pioneer of many forms of outreach clinics for practitioners and students, including a post 9/11 clinic serving rescue teams and their dogs near Ground Zero, and a post—graduate internship serving survivors of sexual assault at a New York City hospital. Prior to studying Chinese Medicine, Kathleen was a performing vocalist of classical music and obtained her BA from Columbia University in Italian Studies.*

Q: How does doing community outreach help students to break down preconceptions and stereotyping?

KG: In health care it is important for students to push beyond familiar interpersonal contacts and gain exposure beyond the known. Health care providers have to treat many different types of individuals and often have no choice in the matter. It is essential to have exposure to the myriad of humanity to prepare to work with human beings of all levels and needs. Community outreach forces students to go beyond the familiar and interact with cultures beyond their own.

As an example, I have supervised students working in HIV/AIDS clinics in New York City. The clinics help students to break down preconceptions and stereotypes related to gender, sexual orientation, economics, race, culture, and chemical dependency. For the majority of students there was some area that was an unknown and therefore a challenge.

Some began to see that HIV/AIDS doesn't just involve the gay male population or drug users, but can be transmitted through heterosexual contact, or contaminated blood transfusions; it can be transmitted by itinerant workers to their spouses at home, or be transmitted by people who refuse to use condoms for cultural or religious reasons. I don't try to influence a change in students' minds, but advise them to focus on the clinical issues when they treat a patient, and to put all personal and judgmental issues aside.

For the most part, the students benefited from their experiences and gained tolerance, patience and understanding. There is an additional benefit; the student may find that through evolved tolerance they will expand their idea of what "type" of patient they are willing to treat. Conversely, community outreach experience helps them to identify future specializations—or—jobs they would prefer to avoid.

It takes a special tolerance and patience to work with chemical dependency issues. Some students find they absolutely cannot work with this population. It's part of their education, knowing what does not work for them as well as what does. Other students find a special talent in dealing with chemical dependency issues, a talent unknown before working in a community/public health care setting.

Another important issue that students learn when working in a community outreach clinic that has a focus on HIV, is the perseverance it takes to work with chronic disease. When a student begins a process of treating with Acupuncture there is the "goal", if you will, of "curing" and the expectation for immediate change. Working with chronic illness requires tenacity because there is no "cure"; there is treatment to slow down the debilitating aspect of the disease, ameliorating medication side effects, keeping the person from developing co-infections and coping with the emotional ups and downs that accompany living with a chronic illness.

Community outreach work also helps students to identify their preference for working in acute—or chronic care—after they graduate. Of course some students will evolve with clinical experience into new areas. I can think of one student who really surprised me. She was very dedicated to the chronic care type of patient while a student. I met her a few years after graduation and she had completely changed course in her Acupuncture work. She found that she lost patience with chronic care so she changed her direction and opened an acute care sports medicine clinic.

Q: You were instrumental in founding the Professional Acupuncture Response Team (PART) after the events of September 11th. Can you describe the evolution of the PART project?

KG: Within the first days post September 11 2001 attack on the World Trade Center, members of the faculty from the Pacific College of Oriental Medicine (PCOM) in New York City were searching for a way to bring Licensed Acupuncturists to Rescue Workers. They landed at the Jacob Javits Center—a large building structure that typically houses conventions on Manhattan's West Side. Post September 11 it was converted to barracks to provide food, shelter and rest for the many Rescue Workers, and dogs, who came to NYC to help search the rubble for human life and to provide protection to the city.

Licensed Acupuncturists were given permission to treat Rescue Workers at the Javits Center. We were committed to 24 hour availability; this was a stipulation of the agreement with federal and state authorities. As I had recently stepped down from a position of President of the Acupuncture Society of NY (ASNY), I got calls from colleagues to help provide leadership for the project. It took quite a bit of coordination to provide the practitioner power to staff a 24 hour mission. PCOM was the first school/organization to staff the project. As the days evolved the other NY Acupuncture schools and professional organizations all contributed to the project. The response of both faculty and students enabled us to maintain the 24 hour on call staffing for the Rescue Workers.

There was a core group of Acupuncturists that participated in the organization of schedules, security issues and solicitations of Asian Medicine companies for all the supplies we needed. The companies showed tremendous generosity and we were well supplied with equipment ranging from tables to needles, Chinese Herbs, massage oils and anything else we required to treat the Rescue Workers.

The core group of individuals would communicate regularly via telephone conference call to keep the organizational flow going and deal with the many issues that arose as we pulled together this amazing project for about four to six weeks. The group eventually came up with the name Professional Acupuncture Response Team, PART.

Q: Can you describe the treatment procedures?

KG: All workers had access to Acupuncture, Massage, Asian Bodywork, Chinese Herbs and Chiropractic services. There were about 20 tables available for treatment at all times and the wait list was always long. Many in our profession have Massage and Asian Bodywork backgrounds and those that did not used their knowledge of the meridians and the body to apply hands-on-healing when needles could not be tolerated. Or, ear needles were inserted as a first foray into Acupuncture together with hands-on Bodywork.

We also treated the rescue dogs. The dogs are specially trained to work in the rubble to search for survivors. In this mission they rarely found anyone alive. This was very depressing for them. They were working very long hours with their trainers and that combined with the disappointment of a perceived "failed" mission made them prime candidates for the healing and caring services we provided. It would often be the case where the trainer was on the table receiving Acupuncture, and the dog was on the floor with a different practitioner, also receiving care, sometimes with needles and many times through healing touch.

We treated hard core, seasoned fire fighters who were receiving Acupuncture for the first time. They were amazed at how effective the treatments were for muscle pain and fatigue, respiratory issues both acute and chronic, stress and strain from the long hours and the emotional impact of the mission. Like the canines, they were also depressed that so few human beings were found alive. Their gratitude was heart warming and memorable to this day.

Q: Did PART survive as an organization?

KG: PART is no longer active. When the Rescue workers were sent home and the Javits Center shut down we continued to work with the local firefighters. Over time the need for PART in NY ended. I do know that there are individuals who continue to work with NY firefighters and programs that grew out of the acute response do continue to offer auricular services.

Q: *What other projects and/or populations have you worked with where Acupuncture is utilized to address crisis and trauma?*

KG: The Tri-State College of Acupuncture (TSCA) in New York recently began an outreach program to create a post-graduate internship to work with survivors of sexual assault at St. Vincent's hospital.

I did volunteer work for 10 years in a rape crisis intervention program in NY at St. Luke's hospital about 12 years ago. I have also treated survivors of sexual assault and incest in my private practice. As such, I was experienced with the population and the staff that serve the population. I was asked to help foster the program and in addition facilitate an informative and treatment based in-service to the volunteers and staff that would be recipients of Acupuncture treatments. The idea was to treat that group first and accustom them to the benefits of the work and iron out the kinks before offering the service to the survivors.

Clearly, this is a population that requires tremendous sensitivity. In this particular setting treating the survivors as a group could possibly help the acceptance of the needles. Needles penetrating the body can be a highly charged treatment for survivors of sexual assault. The insertion of needles can feel like a violation to the hardiest of individuals, so treating someone who has been sexually violated requires mindful care. If a group of individuals with a similar background come together to help each other heal in a safe environment and choose to utilize Acupuncture as part of the process, the co-survivors, along with the Licensed Acupuncturist and experienced staff members, can lend support if the treatment does trigger panic or a sense of being "pinned down."

One of the beauties of Acupuncture is that it can be a non-verbal therapy that allows one to return to a place of health and healing before trauma and can complement the "talk therapy" that also accompanies a healing process. It allows one to reintegrate body with mind and spirit.

Q: *What is an ideal way to prepare students in practical and well informed steps for the many aspects of this work? Sexual assault can*

range from street attack by a stranger, or gang rape to marital or date rape, to incest. How would you advise teachers to prepare their students?

KG: Again, this requires sensitivity and training. Some may think compassion and desire to treat this population is enough but that actually is incorrect. Informed training is key to this work. Also incorrect is the wounded attempting to heal or treat the wounded.

If students or interns have a history with sexual assault either of a personal nature or through a family or a friend's experience, it is very important for them to have the sort of professional interaction they may require to help them process their own experience.

When I was a volunteer at the hospital we had to go through an interview process to screen for readiness to participate in the program. The screening allowed the full time staff to assess whether a person was indeed in a position to advocate for, or work with, survivors without dragging inappropriate baggage into the room. Once this process had been completed and the person cleared to move forward there was a three day training program.

The program included information sessions on the many forms that rape can take. Sexual assault can involve known assailants as well as strangers. It can be extremely violent. In addition to the rape, a person may also incur severe physical damage. It can be the case that a survivor is not being seen for the first time. Rape, contrary to many people's preconceived notions has no gender or age boundaries. Another aspect of discussion is the concept that rape is about sex, this is rarely the case. It is about conflicts with power, dominance, fear, control, and often a perpetrator has been raped or incested themselves.

The best way to prepare a student or postgraduate Acupuncturist to work with this population requires a screening interview conducted by the professional staff trained to work full time with this population as well as a training program as described above. These programs are typically offered as part of a hospital's rape intervention program for volunteers. In addition, the interns need to have ongoing, regularly scheduled supervision with either the clinical staff of the program, or with a Licensed Acupuncturist with a background in treating trauma, particularly sexual trauma.

The initial screening should be done by the hospital staff because they are adept at picking up nuances around this issue that others may not see. In terms of treatment of the population in a community based clinic, I imagine a survivor would be comfortable initially in a peer group setting with appropriate lighting, exits and a minimal amount of needles. Treatment of the extremities and ears with no disrobing is as non-invasive as possible. Listening to the patient is key to helping them regain empowerment.

Allowing them to control the treatment, without disrespect to the provider, also supports empowerment and regaining body control. Control may include requests for a specific practitioner, or rejection of a practitioner related to gender or cultural background, the number of needles used and where.

I recall a patient who as an incest survivor was always approached from the left side by the perpetrator; as a result, for the first few treatments, I could not needle her left side. We worked around this and over time, as she acclimated to the work, we approached the left and began to release the stuck holding patterns.

Practitioners can not personalize the requests and needs of the survivors. However, legitimate requests for comfort and tolerance should be respected and not personalized. As a survivor becomes more comfortable with the experience of Acupuncture and seasoned in the effects, they can model the benefits for new members of the group. This is always far more effective than a practitioner trying to "convince" someone to give it a try.

It is helpful for the recipients of treatment to verbalize or debrief, if you will, post treatment. Sometimes people want to talk and sometimes they will wish for quiet, it is their option. There should always be a trained counselor or therapist "on call" if there is a serious emotional response that occurs due to treatment.

Q: *Similarly, how do you prepare your students to be aware of future patients that may be survivors of such attacks, or in fact, survivors of some form of addiction, details of which may only emerge well into an Acupuncture session or after many sessions?*

KG: I always encourage the students to lean on the supervisory team for the duration of their rotations. There have been numerous occasions over the years in the intern clinic where supervisors have been able to help students navigate flashbacks, aggressive behavior or inappropriately provocative behavior. There is no set approach to managing any of these issues. I encourage the students to set clear boundaries, which feel safe and appropriate for them based on the many discussions they have with faculty over their three years of training. I strongly encourage them not to break their boundaries because the one time they do is when the unexpected emerges. Consistency in behavior creates stability in the practice.

Aggressive behavior can be met with calm and reflective response. Unless one has professional training in counseling or therapy in addition to Acupuncture it can be risky to continue treatment with a patient who continually exhibits aggressive behaviors. In fact the patient may be better served by referral to another practitioner.

Flashbacks can involve tears and emotional releases. It is helpful to assess whether needles need to be removed or not. Often times a cooling cloth on the forehead is helpful and then just sitting and instilling calm into the treatment room can help the patient to return to their own inner calm and body balance. On occasion a gentle touch on the hand or shoulder can ground a person. Other times not making any physical contact is the more appropriate course.

Modeling professional, calm and nonjudgmental or reactive behavior in any challenging clinical interaction is very helpful for students. Explaining choices after the "crisis" is averted is part of their education.

In Supervision sessions students have expressed frustrations with certain types of patients. I try to help them see that if they are that irritated, perplexed or possibly overwhelmed with a patient, they need to seek guidance from a mentor, or possibly, let the patient go, as in refer out. Often these challenging patients can be amazing teaching cases for the entire class, and students evolve a deeper understanding of how to manage, or when to release, a patient.

I encourage students to cultivate a meditation, Tai Chi, Yoga or spiritual practice to ground their own energies. In addition I always encourage them to seek out supervision post-grad, to continue to cultivate information on creative and evolving strategies to deal with the behaviorally and emotionally challenging patients they are bound to meet in practice.

Q: Can you share any surprising instances that arose from your community outreach work that were surprisingly successful or surprisingly disappointing?

KG: I go back to the PART experience. I was surprised and so pleased to see hardened veterans of the armed services and fire departments, 99% male over the age of 45 years, embracing Acupuncture and its healing effects. These men returned for multiple sessions during their mission to New York. They were not immune to the mind, spirit aspect of the work that supported the somatic healing that took place for them.

Q: How do you prepare students to address and avoid compassion fatigue?

KG: It is important to acknowledge that the concept of compassion fatigue is real and it does exist; then to follow up with open and honest discussion about the pitfalls of such fatigue. Of course all health care workers, Acupuncturists included, must walk through a little of the fire. It is hoped that with education they will not be completely burned.

At TSCA I am one of a team of faculty that participates in Supervision. This is a time when students are encouraged to discuss and explore the complex issues of boundaries, compassion fatigue, burnout, population resistance and the like. There is no set course for avoiding compassion fatigue because each individual has to find their limits and work with supervision, practice, time and experience to observe the issues and catch themselves before the fatigue is too deep.

C: LOOKING EAST—FACING WEST

There is no one method for attaining realization of the Tao. To regard any method as the method *is to create a duality, which can only delay your understanding of the subtle truth.*—Lao Tzu *Hua Hu Ching (1)*

We shape clay into a pot. But it is the emptiness inside that holds whatever we want. (verse 11)—Lao Tzu *Tao Te Ching (2)*

WANDERING calligraphy by Yuxia Qiu LAc

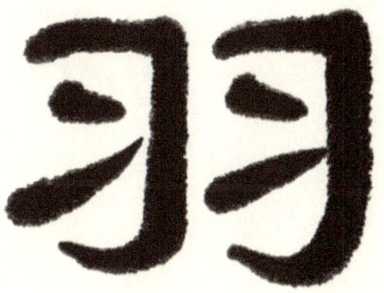

15

Weaving American and Asian Medicine Together

ANNE GRAY BS, RT(T), LAc, MSOM, Dipl OM (NCCAOM), *Austin based Acupuncturist, Herbalist and Feng Shui Consultant, former instructor, Academy of Oriental Medicine, Austin. Former director, School of Radiation Therapy, Department of Radiation Oncology, Memorial Sloan-Kettering Cancer Center, New York City.*

Q: What is the ideal Anatomy and Physiology training for Acupuncture students to help them develop a simultaneous understanding of Western and Asian Medicine?

AG: The primary focus should be hands-on, less book learning, and more emphasis on hands-on-warm-breathing-living bodies. I was a pre-med student which meant extensive cadaver labs. But cadaver labs are of limited learning value for Acupuncture students who would be better served by instructors with great palpation skills. For example, when they learn the *Hara* in a Shiatsu class, it would be great to have someone standing next to them to teach (western) abdominal diagnosis, so they can actually palpate the Liver, Stomach and Spleen organs. When I ran the Radiation Therapy School at Sloan-Kettering, I got more response from my students when I brought them to observe surgery, seeing a living, breathing interior. Similarly when a physician used a scope to diagnose the extent of a tumor on a larynx, they could see the vocal cords in motion, and the extent of the tumor erosion. This made more sense to students (Western or Asian Medicine) than sticking them in a room with a stinky dead body and making them cut it up!

Q: Can you give an example of a dual Western-Asian Medical crossover you shared with students during a class on western diseases?

AG: Breast Cancer! I was able to incorporate the diagnosis of Liver *Qi* Stagnation of Chinese Medicine with the western correlation between breast cancer and Estrogen. The Liver plays a physiological role in the Estrogen cycle in the body. In its original form, Estrogen is sent to the Liver to be conjugated so the body can make full use of it. But if the Liver is being overwhelmed with a difficult job (stress, alcohol, caffeine, or toxins from petroleum plants as in cancer alley of East Texas) it cannot conjugate Estrogen efficiently, so it stores it in breast tissue (where it feeds breast cancer cells). Connections like this help students to appreciate that an understanding of the Western approach to health and illness can make them better practitioners.

Q: What is the ideal Pre-Acupuncture training for students to equip them for a better insight into Western Medicine?

AG: A minimum of high school biology and chemistry, and an undergraduate degree. During their training I would also recommend at least six months of observation in one of the city's free clinics. There they will often see the kind of client who will walk into their student clinic, as well as their private practice. Especially enlightening will be the uninsured and underinsured clients who, because of their situation, will present with full blown symptoms since they were unable to afford preventive or early stage treatment. This will fully immerse students in Western Medicine. I would also encourage schools to employ instructors who fully understand both sides of the fence, Western Medicine and Chinese Medicine, to show students how to think on both sides of the fence to be responsible health care professionals.

Q: How did you teach your students about contraindications between Western Medications and Chinese Herbs?

AG: In my pharmacology classes I told my students they had to think about the typical American patient who is not necessarily encouraged to share all wellness practices with their caregivers because of the judgmental and discouraging response they have received from MDs in the past.

Instead of asking "are you taking supplements?" I sit with my patients and ask them, "What supplements are you taking?" I also asked RNs and Pharmacists for the most commonly prescribed medications (anti-depressants, high blood pressure meds, anti-cholesterol meds). Then I put in extra time in class focusing on the most commonly prescribed medications, and added the Chinese Herbal interactions and contraindications with these specific classes of drugs.

Q: How could clinical training be improved to expand students' awareness of Western diseases?

AG: At a minimum I'd like to see a Nurse Practitioner in each and every student clinic to help with those situations where an immediate need for Western Medical intervention is necessary. There have been recorded instances where Acupuncture students, who were licensed and trained Western Medical professionals, have intervened in such emergencies, as in cases of meningitis, TB and other communicable diseases, as well as myocardial infarction, a non-communicable disease but immediately life threatening. These diagnoses were missed by the Acupuncture clinical supervisors who typically had little Western Medical training.

Ideally I would also like to see a clinical practicum offered in the final year of training where patients with active Western diagnoses who need Western Medical care, would be brought in to help students understand when they need to make referrals, and when Chinese Herbs could have serious contraindications with their Western medications.

Q: How did you expand students' awareness of Public Health issues?

AG: Public Health was one of the classes I enjoyed teaching the most. Each week every student was assigned to bring to class a current news report directly related to sickness and health, preferably, in their local community. We would then spend the first hour of each three-hour class discussing the ramifications of these stories. This raised their community awareness, and trained them to monitor health trends for the benefit of their future patients. What I wanted them to understand was where they fit into the health system of the USA. One student went above and beyond her peers on the subject of childhood obesity and its possible link to increased diabetes. She called all the schools in the area to track the connection between school menus and childhood obesity. So I knew that when she had a patient—perhaps a kid with a serious case of childhood obesity—she wouldn't just treat is as a *Damp Phlegm* problem. She would also sit and talk to the patient and the parents about the role of proper nutrition in their own and their child's present and future health.

Q: Share some stories with us of the mistakes you've observed in both Chinese and Western Medicine?

AG: When I worked at Sloan—Kettering in Radiation Oncology, we were treating a patient for lung cancer and started to notice that he was having a severe skin reaction early on in his course of treatment. Any patient receiving radiation therapy has to be very careful with skin care because the skin becomes more sensitive to sun and heat. We were concerned when we started to notice his burns. Only then he told us he was seeing a Chinese Herbalist in Chinatown who was using herbal plasters on his chest regularly. We told him he must stop applying the herbal heated plasters immediately. Also we had to discontinue his radiation treatments for a while which probably compromised his long-term outcome.

On the other side of the fence, I was able to solve the medical mystery surrounding a client's husband who had suffered a retinal hemorrhage. Even though I had never examined him, I knew of his continuing cardiac problems because of my discussions with his wife. This was a major source of stress in her life, especially because he was on Coumadin, a very strong blood thinner. When she arrived in my office after leaving him in hospital, we spent some time discussing his case. I asked her if his Coumadin levels were regularly monitored. She said they were but he had been having difficulties keeping it balanced over the past several months, a problem that stymied his physicians. I knew from my intake with her that she was using over-the-counter supplements on a daily basis, including Vitamin E, Garlic and Gingko Biloba, all of which affect the blood's ability to clot. I asked if her husband was taking the same supplements (he was) and whether he had informed his physicians (which he had not). Through my urging she did report this to his MD who took immediate action to resolve the situation. Ironically, she would not tell the MD that it was her *Acupuncturist* who solved the mystery!

Patients sometimes get overwhelmed with intake forms, and so they rush through them. I spend at least 20 minutes taking a client through the intake forms. From day one, I ask them about supplements, as well as prescription and illegal drug use. An honest exchange of information is crucial. A lot of patients are scared of telling their MDs they are on Chinese Herbs, or any type of care not specifically prescribed by an MD.

In another case I had a client with high blood pressure and high cholesterol, who had been taking Western medications for six years without much success. She was also suffering from lower body edema. When I did not see the expected response I reviewed her prescription drugs thoroughly. Her high BP medication was directly responsible for her edema. I adjusted my prescription accordingly and resolved the situation. I also asked her what she had eaten over the last three days and was horrified by her daily consumption of fast food. I gave her a healthier eating plan which, in six years of Western Medical care, no one had ever discussed with her!

Q: How can such basic mistakes be avoided?

AG: My ideal would be a multidisciplinary clinic where practitioners, MDs, Chiropractors, Nutritionists, Naturopaths and Acupuncturists would work side-by-side, take apart and share case studies. Acupuncturists are so busy trying to be mini-doctors they do a disservice to their clients and the disciplines of Asian Medicine. We need to teach students that MDs are not the enemy and that there are limitations to Chinese Medicine as well. Some students even ask why they need to study Western Medicine! Well, by showing them we have taken the time to learn and to understand Western Medicine and "speak their language" we validate them and their profession, and hopefully plant the seed for them to do the same for us. How can we expect Western Medical practitioners to accept us as professionals and colleagues if we do not accord them the same respect?

Pam and Debra's footnote: We're sad to report that shortly after Annie Gray completed her conversations with us, she died suddenly in Austin, Texas on July 27, 2007. An outspoken New Yorker of Irish and Lithuanian ancestry, Annie will always be remembered as a teacher who used storytelling to weave her years of hospital expertise in America into the fabric of Asian Medicine in a colorful and practical way.

16

Theater and Therapists—
Developing Interaction Skills

MEGAN COLE, MA *Actor of Stage and TV, created the leading role in the Pulitzer Prize winning play WIT which she has performed at theaters on the West Coast and in the Southwest. Her many TV roles include Seinfeld, The Practice, Judging Amy, Star Trek, L.A. Law, and ER (where she plays the role of the pathologist). As a result of her role in WIT she was invited to be Artist-in-Residence at the University of Texas at Houston's Health Science Center, to develop courses in physician-patient interaction skills for medical, nursing, dental and research students.*

Q: How did your role in WIT, and especially your observations during post performance discussions with audiences, oncologists, and cancer survivors, alert you to problems in physician/patient interaction skills?

MC: After performances of WIT, audience members would frequently come to me, in person or by mail, to say how much the experience of the play had meant to them. "I feel as if I'm able to mourn my grandmother for the first time," one woman said. "My wife died of cancer six months ago," a young man wrote, "and in some way I don't understand, the play is helping me accept her loss." "God, this was *exactly* my experience," exclaimed many cancer survivors, "I'm so glad to be given a voice."

But what I repeatedly noted was that many *doctors* who saw the play had a very different reaction. "Well," they'd say, "it's a fine play, but you know, the reality of doctor/patient relationships is nothing like that." And that disparity of perception between patients and physicians led me to wonder if there might be something from my acting knowledge that might be useful in narrowing that gap.

Q: UT Houston/Health Science Center invited you to teach special electives in physician/patient interaction skills on the strength of the WIT dynamic. How did you structure these workshops using "acting models"?

MC: In my course, variously titled "The Craft of Empathy," "Developing the Skills of Conscious Equanimity," and "Balancing Engagement and Detachment," I draw on actors' skills for being both inside and outside a character at the same moment.

One of the things I hear most often from doctors is the fear that if they become too emotionally involved with their patients, they risk losing their professional objectivity. So what I try to suggest is that when we make *conscious choices* about our behavior and have techniques for balancing our involvement and non-involvement (which is, of course, what actors do), the fear of losing the Self in the Other is greatly diminished, because we are in control at all times.

I structure my sessions around both *skills* and *principles,* all drawn from actors' techniques.

The *skills* include:

- Identifying the inner witness,
- Using conscious breathing,
- Behaving "as if",
- Analyzing content through action/objective/obstacle,
- Becoming aware of the role of status in the communication encounter,
- Developing awareness of subtext and nonverbal signals,
- Becoming aware of context, or "given circumstances."

The *principles* include: Balance, Equanimity, Awareness, Choice, Empathy, Compartmentalizing, Perspective, Self-Monitoring, Focus, and Intention. Each class is a combination of:

- My talking about and demonstrating these principles and skills, along with—
- Some interactive exercises and group discussion.

I try to avoid being too didactic or academic, and focus instead on a *balance* of emotional engagement and intellectual detachment with the students, so that the class itself is a model of the subject matter.

Q: What sort of feedback do you get from medical, dental and nursing students after these electives?

MC: Each series concludes with a brief written evaluation from the students, who answer questions about what they liked most about the classes and what they think needs improvement. From the evaluations that I've seen (and perhaps I've only been shown the good ones!), the responses have been very positive. Overall, what they seem most to have appreciated is that they get nothing else like this in their medical training. And the most repeated request for improvement is to have relatively more discussion. I hear them.

Q: Do they enjoy the role-playing aspect of the exercise—and can you give some concrete examples?

MC: I don't do role-playing per se, as in, "You be the doctor and someone else will be the patient." I do, though, use various interactive exercises. To give you a couple of examples:

- When we're talking about Behaving "As If," I will ask a couple of students to describe themselves using 2 adjectives, then ask them to tell us, say, what they had for breakfast as if they were the *opposite* of those qualities.

- Using parts of scenes from WIT, I will ask for a volunteer to work with me to read the lines using different actions, objectives, and obstacles, or

- Different subtexts, or

- Different given circumstances, or

- Different status.

- We always work on diaphragmatic breathing, which is so fundamental to balance.

- When talking about nonverbal signals, I might ask them to, say, cock their heads to one side and then try to feel authoritative, or to frown and say "I love you" without irony.

These kinds of exercises have proved popular and (I believe) instructive, even though it's not easy getting medical students to volunteer.

Q: During your talk at a school of Acupuncture, you quoted the same line of text in three very different voices to highlight the importance of observing patients' body language, and listening to tone and texture, beyond mere words. Can you quote the sentence and the very different meanings you conveyed through tone?

MC: The passage is: "I don't mean to complain, but I am becoming very sick. Very, very sick. Ultimately sick, as it were." These are just words on a page until we consider the subtext—what we really mean underneath the words we say. So I changed the underlying thought—the attitude—three times and asked the students to watch body language and tone of voice. The three tones were:

- Angry ("This is all your fault"),
- Sad ("I'm going to die and I'm not ready"), and
- Defended ("Hey, this is no big deal").

Q: Can you repeat the source that inspired this exercise?

MC: Dr. Albert Mehrabian, professor emeritus at UCLA, published a classic text (1) on nonverbal communication in 1972. His studies showed that the messages we send are composed of these parts: 55% body language, 38% tone of voice, and 7% words. Thus, *how* we say something outweighs *what* we say by about nine to one.

Q: You also spoke about the importance of physicians/therapists using acting techniques/self centering techniques as preparation for working with patients, especially very complex patients. Can you give some examples? Many physicians are criticized for the clumsy ways in which they inform patients & families about terminal illness. Did you role play life/death topics, and did students tell you that your workshops were the first to help them practice those interaction skills?

MC: I believe the most important of the centering techniques is *witnessing*—an identification with the part of the self that is *not* involved in the emotion of whatever is currently happening.

An example I might use is: You might tell me you're feeling depressed. I'd ask, "Have you been noticing the depression more lately?" and you might answer, "Yes, I have." At that point I'd say, "Is whoever it is that is noticing this, *also* depressed?" In other words, when you say, "I'm depressed," who is the "I" who is saying this? Who is the "I" who is objective enough to stand apart and notice you're depressed? That self who is noticing is the witness, the observer. (I have adapted this example from Dr. Wayne Dyer; I also use examples from my acting.) My overall point is that we can, by conscious choice, move between states of mind, and that when we know we can do that, we're in control of our behavior.

I don't specifically address the issue of breaking bad news, largely because I have no personal experience doing this. I do suggest that the techniques we're working with can certainly be useful in life/death discussions with patients and families, as in less dire encounters. My impression is that the vast majority of the students I've met have had zero training in breaking bad news. *Aaarrggh!*

Q: How seriously was your work as artist-in-residence taken by members of the medical school faculty? How did you overcome skepticism?

MC: It's uphill all the way to get my work taken seriously by any but a few members of the medical school faculty. The course is an elective, not a requirement. Lunch, that crucial lure, is not served. A single faculty member might wander into a session or two, but I have no sense that my work is anywhere on their radar screens—it's seen rather as peripheral fluff for which there is no time in an overcrowded curriculum.

My guess is I *might* be taken more seriously if I had a PhD after my name, if I were not an actor, and/or if I were Meryl Streep, i.e., famous. As it is, I'm some nutty act*ress* who shows up occasionally to soothe a few students' flagging idealism with new-age blather about compassion and stuff. My work is very marginalized—except, I believe, with a majority of the students who are actually brave enough to take the series.

For a couple of years I tried to deal with skepticism by making my classes somewhat more "intellectual"—I started writing lists on the blackboard, for example, and making up mnemonics for remembering lists—but soon realized that since I am after all, for better or worse, an actor, I need to stay close to what

I know best, which is to move people emotionally, and to know *how* to do that in a consistent manner. My strength is that I *am* an actor, nutty or not, who thinks that idealism is a good thing, that empathic skills can be taught, and that the body and the mind do in fact work in concert. Radical stuff, but probably worth fighting for.

Q: Several medical schools (Yale, Stanford, Cornell, Mt Sinai, among others) are introducing art-appreciation classes to help develop students' observation skills. Ideally, how could such courses be expanded to include your electives in the performing arts?

MC: I'd like to see medical schools present a package of arts-related opportunities for students, as if, imagine, we were not competing with each other. Why not combine viewing great museum art with exploring great plays and great operas and even great medically-related movies and TV shows? UT has an annual program called "Healthcare and the Arts," which is a wonderful idea and which is generally ignored by the medical school population. You can't legislate people's interests, but perhaps you can convince them that spending a little time with the arts might be in their best interests. How to do that is the question.

Q: How have your workshops evolved/changed during each year at UT Houston? And what have you observed/learned about gaps in standard medical education?

MC: When I first created the course in 2000, my proposed title was "The Other Self: The Experience of Empathy." That was rejected as being too vague and mystifying for medical students, but it's actually what I mean: we can only begin to understand what it's like to be another person when we relate their experience to our own. So I changed the title that first year to "Empathic Communication with Patients," and it's pretty much been a variation of that until this year, when it became "Balancing Engagement and Detachment."

In general, the arc of the six years I've been doing this work has been a refining of the material—to zero in on what in fact I mean to say and to drop things that might sound good but are actually peripheral. The idea of using actors' techniques in medical training seems to be fairly unique, meaning, on the simplest level, there is no material out there for me to crib, paraphrase, steal, or otherwise appropriate!

I do less of my own acting now, preferring to use the time to (try to) involve the students. I've dropped an entire session on empathic listening, since a respected mentor pointed out I didn't have the requisite hundreds of hour listening to patients. I've stopped using actual acting improvisations with these students, since they simply don't have the background to make the exercises useful, or to overcome their fear. I've deleted the session on literature and medicine, as being way too large to handle in such a short time (I do, though, conduct a whole separate series on this subject). And the content is in general somewhat more objective and happens to be less philosophical.

I believe the course in its present incarnation is tighter, more to the point, more take-home useful—and because it's less overtly "dramatic," probably a little less riveting.

As for gaps in medical education, my observation is the obvious: a severe over-reliance on technology at the sad expense of hands-on, human-oriented health-care. This is axiomatic, but even with the occasional arts or communication class, not much is being done about it.

Q: And on that basis, what new themes are you exploring for future workshops?

MC: I'm presently looking into doing a series on Medical Readers' Theater, based on a program developed at the East Carolina University's Brody School of Medicine, and published in a guide edited by Todd L. Savitt. (2) The concept involves adapting short stories about medicine to scripts and giving them public readings with medical students as the "actors," followed by discussions with the audience. This format might be good for actively involving the students in their education, and for creating a dialogue about important ethical and social issues in medicine.

On the first and last days of the course, I confess to the students that the series is a little more subversive than its title suggests. It's really about asking, "Who do I want to be?" and then looking for answers that are slightly outside the box.... .

17

The Prisms of Clinical Counseling and Communication

Lorena Monda LAc, OMD, MS *New Mexico based Acupuncturist, Body-Centered Psychotherapist, and Qigong instructor. She is the author of "The Practice of Wholeness: Spiritual Transformation in Everyday Life" (1) and, with John Scott, has also co-authored the "Clinical Guide to Commonly Used Chinese Herbal Formulas"(2). She teaches Asian Medicine and Psychology, Clinical Counseling and Communication Skills.*

Q: Did you complete your formal training in psychology before your Acupuncture training—or after? And why?

LM: I trained in Psychology before I went to Acupuncture school. At the time, there was little about the body in Psychology. I became interested in Asian Medicine after studying Tai Chi back in the early 80s, and then having a pivotal experience with one of my counseling clients—a 17-year-old boy who ended up in a coma after brain surgery. This experience made me look for a system of working with the body that had potential for linking the body and mind. I was only 25 years old and working in a family therapy program, which also had a peer-counseling component for young people. My client, John, was in the hospital in a coma. The hospital was directly on my way home from work, so I would visit him every day, sit with him, hold his hand and talk to him. After about a month of this, I was invited to a staff meeting to discuss his case with the head neurosurgeon, his nurses, and social worker. The head neurosurgeon asked me who I was, and what I was doing there. When I told him I was John's counselor, he told me I was wasting my time because the patient would always be a vegetable.

This made me furious. When I left the meeting, I went back into John's room, held his hand and told him about the meeting and what was said there. I told him that I didn't believe the doctor's prognosis; I didn't believe he would never come out of the coma. I was running on my instincts at this point. I said to him, "I believe you have a choice"—and at that moment he squeezed my hand. I told him that recovery might be hard, but whatever it took—I would help him—and he squeezed my hand again. He did eventually regain consciousness and went on to live a normal life. This whole experience changed my life. I started reading everything I could find about body-mind and alternative healing, started taking Tai Chi—I was in Los Angeles at the time, studied at the Taoist Institute, went on a spiritual journey to Mexico. I went to massage school and then trained in Asian Medicine.

Q: Do you share this story with your students as a way of emphasizing the body-mind connection?

LM: Yes, and other stories as well. I want to help students to develop instinctive ways of working with patients, to use their intuition. I have many stories like this. Another pivotal case for me was that of a patient who had chronic Kidney Yin and Yang deficiency to the point of chronic fatigue. She had been to many practitioners. I had been taught to take pulses at the beginning and at the end of a session. I would treat this patient and she would feel better for a day or three days, then her Kidney energy would crash back down again. I got the bright idea to take pulses in the *middle* of the treatment and ask her as I felt her energy coming back up, "what are you experiencing now?" She had a memory of being in her house as a child, being really excited and having a lot of energy and her mother constantly asking her to calm down because her dad was suffering from a heart ailment. And so as her energy would come up she had this message in her psyche that said, you can't feel this good, you can't be excited, you can't have this energy because your dad will die. So it was nearly impossible, until we discovered that, for her to have energy. We could have done Acupuncture and herbs forever and never discovered that. The essential thing was her bringing consciousness to the feeling of having more energy, what that was like for her, and what came up for her as she experienced herself with energy. That was how we discovered a little piece of information that was essential to her healing. Then little by little, this patient could work with her *Qi* in present time. I asked her if her father was still alive, she said no. "Then you can't kill him by having energy." This patient taught me to work with the direct experience of *Qi* in present time.

Our *Qi* is held by our thoughts, our emotions, and our experiences. If we work with *Qi* as a direct experience, we can train our patients to track their own *Qi*. Many students get panicked, thinking this is psychotherapy, but it isn't. This is working with *Qi*. This, I tell my students, is what treatments are all about, not only about methodology and needle technique, but about being clear and mindful in the treatment process, and helping the patient get mindful as well so that they can affect their own healing.

Q: How do you teach students to deal with aggressive patients?

LM: Practitioners should not be afraid of a patient's aggression. It is *Qi* and *Qi* itself is non-pathological, it only becomes pathological when it is used in a way that is not functional. Aggression is a type of *Qi* that serves us sometimes. But I might tell the patient that it doesn't serve them if they are aggressive towards someone trying to treat them. I teach students to contact what is arising directly with the patient. So if aggression is arising, the practitioner can contact it—can say to the patient "do you notice what you are feeling right now?" The patient can be helped to discover what the real function of that *Qi* is and learn to allow the *Qi* to move in a healthy way. I remind students to expect patients to behave like patients. For example a patient might forget their checkbook every week and that is part of their pattern. It doesn't help to blame patients for bringing in such symptoms. We are always trying to balance the ideal against reality. Our job is to act like practitioners, we are in charge of what happens in our treatment session, and we can manage our treatments without blaming patients for having the symptoms.

Q: Ideally, how many hours of training in psychology and psychosocial topics should students receive, and do you feel such topics are generally underserved/neglected by schools of Asian Medicine?

LM: You know, I don't know if it is a question of hours. Students seem overwhelmed by the number of hours they are now required to take. I think that psychology, and the behavioral aspect of medicine—health psychology, should be woven into the curriculum, so that it is not a separation. I think the understanding of these issues is inherent in our medicine, but underdeveloped in the materialistic way the medicine is often taught and practiced.

Q: Do you feel students should also intern in safe havens, refugee centers, homeless shelters, drug and alcohol rehab, psychiatric hospital outpatient units, prisons, juvenile rehab center, etc., to give them a broader view of the community and the wider effects of social stress on health and sanity?

LM: Since part of my initial training was in community/clinical psychology, I am a big believer in the part that social, societal and environmental stress play on physical and mental health. I think that volunteering in community health settings is great, but only if the students are trained to understand the context for what they are doing in these settings. Otherwise it can be overwhelming, and sometimes turns students off.

Q: What subjects do you highlight in your psych classes?

LM: Because I have such a limited time with students (four six-hour classes) I focus on some very basic things:

Class 1: Understanding the psycho-spiritual development and transformation in terms of the Five Phases. We also use this map to deconstruct the emotions in terms of function, *Qi* and, psychological development and family and cultural learning.

Class 2: Basic Psychological Life Questions.

Classes 3–4: These classes are taught to more advanced students with actual treatment experience. The role of presence in communication, and how the practitioners' attitudes affect the communication process. In short, it's an advanced version of the basic skill of reflective listening.

I give them what I call a *Skills Prism*:

1. *Presence and Mindfulness* is on top.

2. *Tracking*—using our senses to track what is going on in the patient's body, emotions, mind, spirit—is on the left.

3. *Contact*—verbally letting the patient know what we are tracking—is on the right.

4. *Directing Awareness* is on the base of the prism—using questions and directives to direct patient's awareness to the present experience, includ-

ing learning how to convert what we are witnessing into a direct experience of *Qi.*

Each of these four skills is connected to each other, they build upon each other.

Then I teach the students what I call *Deconstructing the Treatment Process*—Breaking down the treatment process so students can be clear about some of the basic elements of the treatment process like gathering data and making therapeutic interventions. If students know clearly what entails making therapeutic interventions (with their *Qi* and communication, as well as with needles, Bodywork and Herbs) and how to get the patient more onboard in this process then the treatment becomes vastly more effective. Having the patient onboard empowers patients and increases their understanding and compliance.

Q: How do you teach them to recognize the subtle undercurrents of depression/emotional/psychic stress not often apparent in standard diagnostic methods (tongue/pulse etc)?

LM: By working with direct experience, the subtle undercurrents come quickly to the surface. Also by showing the students the direct relationship between emotions, thoughts, attitudes, beliefs, personal experience, and physical symptoms.

Q: Do you get your students to role-play real life scenarios re therapist-patient encounters to help them address the above issues?

LM: I don't use role playing per se. We work directly with each other using our direct experience. I demonstrate this with them, and I let them practice the skills on me, so that they can see what the process looks like on someone who had been trained to work with her own direct experience and because I can manage the process. Plenty of material comes up from this for teaching about what will happen in the clinic. "We are our patients" is what I tell them. Also I want to break down the wall between patient and practitioner as expert. I want to demonstrate the power of the collaborative process and the benefit of really being transparent in the relationship with our patients. During a sample demonstration, the group acts as the practitioner. I sit in a chair and the students encircle me. I begin with something physical such as a pain in my stomach and they use the "Skills Prism" that they are learning. The students begin with the physical symptom and then use the skills to connect the symptom with other aspects of my experience that they are tracking in the present moment.

Q: Can you tell us more about the "Skills Prism"?

LM: Some other ways I work with the skills include:

1. *Presence*—how to be present without an attitude, or be present and know what attitude you are bringing, i.e., bring an attitude of open curiosity. Students work with partners who tell a story of something mildly challenging in their lives. First the listener gets a baseline of how they normally listen—what are their impulses, what do they want to do as they listen. Then I have them try on different attitudes and listen from there tracking what happens in their bodies, and *Qi* as they listen from these attitudes. Some familiar attitudes are: "there is a problem, and it is my job to fix it" or "this patient is difficult". Then I ask students to listen from the attitude of "this person is an inspiration" and to see how listening affects their body, mind and *Qi*.

2. *Tracking*—through the skill of tracking, we learn to track voice tone, body posture, story, etc., but we can track things in more detail because the unconscious is showing itself through more things—physical and nonphysical. If the patient tells a story and then gets animated, or they pull back, then that tells you something.

3. *Contact*—the students track and name what they track. e.g., "I notice when you said that you really pulled back; did you notice that?"

4. *Directing Awareness*—Students learn to turn their awareness and the patient's awareness toward direct experience, e.g., "How does your stomach feel right now? What kind of ache is that? Are there any emotions that go with that feeling in your stomach?" Then track what's happening as the patient talks about the stomachache. Slow the process so the patient stays on board. The patient can feel the emotion and feel the stomachache. The patient feels the connection directly. Then when the needles shift the energy for the patient and the patient feels better, we can track and inquire "what does feeling better feel like, what is exactly happening when you feel better?" Patients get off the table, we say "how are you feeling?" They say "better" but we never inquire as to what better feels like for them. This information is immensely valuable in help-

ing us understand what needs to happen for that patient, and in helping the patient to have the building blocks for recreating that experience for him or herself.

Q: Do you teach your students to recognize the first signs of Transference?

LM: I used to do this when I had an ethics component in my class. Now what I do is really demonstrate the power of the therapeutic relationship and ways to make this relationship more respectful in terms of boundaries both the patients' boundaries and the practitioners'. I also do a brief (depending on the class, sometimes more extensive) teaching on how to make some of the dynamics more explicit so the patient can be more empowered to find what they need in their lives. I actually spend more time on countertransference and the attitudes we have toward our patients and how they gets in the way of the treatment process. I think it is valuable to teach students how to monitor and adjust their own feelings, attitudes, and beliefs about patients in terms of the transference/countertransference issue. I think transference gets out of control when the practitioner is not mindful of his or her own boundaries and limits.

Q: Do you give your students the guidelines they will need in a future practice re the appropriate time to refer patients to a psychologist/or psychotherapist?

LM: Not in any systematized way (e.g., no handouts) but this always comes up and we spend a lot of time talking about it. I talk about it mostly in the context of internal and external resources, and how to access these resources in ourselves and in our patients. How to assess our and our patients' internal resources for dealing with what is in front of us. And how to use the wonderful myriad of external resources currently available. I give many examples of when I refer to people with more skills than me, when necessary, and of working in collaboration with other practitioners.

Q: What guidelines do you give students who may encounter suicidal patients?

LM: I give basic guidelines on how to assess risk, legal considerations, and the importance of linking the patient with the appropriate mental health resources and hotlines or to call in other resources when necessary.

Q: What do you feel is the most appropriate/diplomatic way of helping students navigate sensitive cross-cultural issues related to the different ways in which instructors or patients from different backgrounds or ethnic groups handle problems related to depression, stress, emotional pain, and abuse issues according to cultural taboos and denials?

LM: I love this topic. I talk a lot about how our experience is mediated by family learning and culture, and how this affects our *Qi*. When we are working in the class, because we have students from other cultures, this comes up directly, and so we address it directly when it does. I talk about becoming curious about differences and also finding commonality in our experiences. I also mention things like historical trauma, war and stress and how that effects health, as it seems to now be a relevant topic in the post-9/11 USA. (Something that people from most other cultures can relate to more easily.)

Q: Do you believe it would be beneficial for students to partake in psychotherapy during the course of their training to address any unresolved issues that might manifest in their future professional encounters? Would you advocate this as a requirement prior to graduation?

LM: I do believe it is beneficial but I am not sure it can be required. I think what might be more effective is to have mentorship/support groups required to get through the education process with someone trained to assess what the student needs psychologically and refer when necessary. I strongly believe that healers develop mastery by working on themselves, by understanding the transformation process from the inside out.

Q: How, if at all, do you address the issue of compassion fatigue and burnout among practitioners in the helping professions?

LM: Burnout is a big issue that always comes up. Students are often burned out by the end of their training. I address it by talking about Yin and nourishment, and the barriers we have to nourishment. We talk about what it takes to be present as a practitioner—what are expectations are about ourselves as practitioners ("a good practitioner is someone who …"). Accepting the reality that we are affected by our patients and learning how to best deal with that reality. I talk a lot about having to keep oneself in the loop as a practitioner, and how to do that in a non-narcissistic way when working with others. If you are giving, giving, giving, all the time and not receiving, your psyche knows this and it will let you know about the imbalance somehow. Health is about *Qi* and *Qi* exchange.

18

Ethics, Borders and Boundaries

CHERIE SOHNEN-MOE, BA (Psychology) *and healing arts practitioner is President of Sohnen-Moe Associates, Inc. She serves on the board of the Arizona School of Acupuncture and Oriental Medicine in Tucson, AZ and is an adjunct professor at the Clayton College of Natural Health. She received the Outstanding Instructor Award from the Desert Institute of the Healing Arts. She is the author of "Business Mastery" (1) and co-author of "The Ethics of Touch"(2). She is a frequent contributor to Massage and Bodywork journals, and a popular presenter at national conventions of Complementary and Alternative Medicine. Cherie serves on the Massage and Bodywork Licensing Exam of the FSMTB.*

Q: Your great work "The Ethics of Touch" co-written with Ben Benjamin PhD contains many examples from different Bodywork Therapies and Acupuncture. What has prompted the most response?

CS-M: We have received a lot of positive feedback. Some say that our explanations of transference, countertransference and boundaries are the best they've ever seen!

Generally training in this area is inadequate in most schools, especially in Acupuncture schools. Transference does not have to be negative—in psychology it is used as a tool. But in Asian Medicine, transference can happen because it is so intimate. I am more worried about countertransference—what the practitioner is feeling rather than what the client is feeling. Practitioners untrained in countertransference don't even recognize it when it happens to them. I am constantly in their faces about how they have to take the time to educate themselves—especially in the Bodywork world. A lot of schools use our *Ethics of Touch* throughout the curriculum—not just in Ethics classes.

Chapter Five has stirred up the most controversy. I am not at all surprised as it's about sex, touch and intimacy. One instructor told us he wasn't even able to access that chapter's online teaching material because it had the word "sex" in it!

The topic is loaded and layered on so many complex levels. I have been working with practitioners who are not traditionally considered to be in the "touch" professions like Pilates, Alexander Technique and Yoga—and this is one of toughest challenges. Practitioners can believe their intention is enough—but if the client has been abused—even the most minimal or well intentioned touch can trigger a flashback. For instance, I am also a rebirther, and made the mistake of placing a bolster under the legs of one of my clients without first asking her. Her feet shot up off the table when her legs were touched in this altered state because she experienced a flashback. Fortunately I knew how to handle the situation—but many therapists would not know how to provide a safe and structured space, and patients could easily become unglued. Sensitivity training is essential for anyone involved in touch therapies.

Q: Do you feel schools of Acupuncture, and Asian Bodywork give sufficient training in the details of Ethics you outline in your book, namely Boundary issues, Business Ethics, and Awareness of underlying complexities like Trauma and PTSD? Most of us learned the hard way when we confronted such situations during years of clinical practice. What would be the ideal training Program? To invite practitioners from the field to share case studies for students to role play?

CS-M: The ideal training would be to address the issues that are in my book. Have the students read the material and initiate class discussions. Do role plays and simulations. Bring in graduate panels so students can ask questions.

Q: How can schools deal with problems of plagiarism?

CS-M: By preventing them before they happen, by writing clear guidelines in the instructors' manual and the students' manual. Unfortunately some teachers set a poor example by giving handouts to students without referencing the source of the material. Teachers do this all the time, freely copying material without asking permission. It's not appropriate, and it makes students think it's OK, and that's how they learn a lack of respect. Schools need to set a climate. Blatant copyright infringement is unacceptable. Schools also need to know that they are liable and could be sued. I talk about this in every teachers' training workshop.

Q: How can schools deal in a sensitive but practical way with "problem" students?

CS-M: Again, there needs to be a clear protocol for students and for teachers, built into the orientation package. There needs to be a system of specific report forms enabling everyone to document incidents or concerns, anonymously if necessary, so there is a paper trail in the case of students causing concerns in different classes. For instance, a teacher might think the behavior is an isolated event and dismiss it. But if multiple reports are filed by different people, then this cues the administration that action needs to be taken. Guidelines should always be included in teachers' training. Teachers—especially new or young teachers—need sensitivity training, and need to know how to take a student aside if necessary, and ask "how is your behavior helpful to your learning?" And every school needs a qualified counselor on staff.

Q: Can you share some examples of how you worked with problem students in your own classes?

CS-M: In one of the schools where I taught a class in communications, I had to work with a student with abrasive behavioral problems—she was a transplant from the east coast to the southwest—and a lot of people had problems with her, and with the language she used. No one wanted to work with her or sit next to her. Students *and* faculty had problems with her. I knew she wasn't a bad person and she didn't want to be disliked. So I asked her permission to see if she wanted to explore the problem in front of the class, using the communication techniques I had been teaching. She agreed, and she was open to hearing feedback from the class. I didn't want to run this like a psychotherapy session. But after the session there was a change in the class, and a change in her. One time, I had two students who were constantly in each other's faces. So I said: "You two need to take this out of class—and don't return until you have sorted this out and can be civil." They returned after an hour.

Then I broke the class into groups and put them together in a "conflict resolution" group. It worked. I wasn't going to abandon them. But I had Rules.

In the first day of a course I also have the class set rules that they want to make the learning environment safe and enjoyable. At this point we also decide how to handle it if someone breaks the rules. Some students are not too fond of me in the first couple of weeks because I have strong expectations of them in terms of personal responsibility—plus I assign a lot of homework—but they are always thankful at the end. And I always get excellent evaluations.

Q: How would you advise teachers in situations where an ethical clash arose because of a cultural misunderstanding? For example, a new teacher or practitioner from one of the Asian countries who was not fully informed about draping requirements in the USA. Or, a situation where a client insisted on, say, a neck adjustment from an Acupuncturist or an Asian Bodywork Therapist in the USA because of receiving such techniques in China or Japan even though this is beyond the scope of practice in the USA.

CS-M: It's very important to learn cultural differences. As a professional—it behooves you to learn about the other culture. Maybe the licensing boards should require practitioners from other countries to study guidelines, to answer exam questions about scope of practice, and boundary issues. First of all, there really is no excuse for practitioners not knowing their professional guidelines and legalities (as in the draping example). The second example is about communication. If a client wants something that the practitioner can't do because of his/her scope of practice, s/he simply needs to say something along the lines of, "I am sure that you benefited from that procedure in country X. Unfortunately, it is illegal for me to do that here." Another option is, "I am sure that you benefited from that procedure. Unfortunately, I am not trained to do those types of procedures."

Q: Let's say an executive received "additional intimate services" in a hotel spa while on business in another country. A month later the executive refused to pay a bone fide practitioner who stopped the session because "additional intimate services" were requested. What would you advise the practitioner to do? Invoice the executive with a lawyer's letter? Or chalk it up to experience and be doubly careful about the specific terminology used to describe the form of therapy to prospective clients over the phone, and in brochures?

CS-M: First of all, why terminate the session? I suggest the practitioner politely yet unapologetically say, "That is totally inappropriate." Now, if the client continues on or becomes offensive, then the practitioner needs to stop the session. Immediately. I would attempt to obtain payment right then. If not, send a bill, but don't put much energy into collection.

I think that it's wise to for brochures to include something along the lines of "What to Expect" to describe the flow of the sessions.

As far as telephone screening, you always want to ask the caller the following:

- What s/he is hoping to get from the work (make sure it's aligned with what you do);

- Has s/he had this type of work before? If so, where, when, and how often? Ask the caller what a typical session was like;

- Then you can say, "Here's how we would work together. The first session consists of.... Subsequent sessions....";

- Ask if s/he has any questions. State your basic policies (fees, cancellation policy, eating a light meal beforehand, etc.); and

- Then book the appointment (or send literature).

Q: What advice do you give practitioners who fall in love with a patient or vice versa? To refer the patient to a colleague immediately? If the feeling is mutual, how many months should the individuals wait between the end of the therapy and the start of a new relationship?

CS-M: Falling in love might be more in the countertransference area. My book offers useful checklists of questions for practitioners who are unclear or confused about their feelings for a patient, and how to handle such situations in a professional and subtle way.

I researched all the state massage board licensing regulations and while they all had strictures against sexual involvement with current clients, only four of them said anything about not dating/having sex with a former client. An interesting case came up in Minnesota where a therapist and former client became roommates, started dating and then married, but didn't wait the required two years.

The client's former wife filed a complaint. Ultimately the case was dropped, but it took a long time and thousands of dollars in legal fees. Physicians, on the other hand, can date a patient the moment they stop treating him/her. That's scary given the potential for such an extreme power differential.

Q: Many practitioners don't know where to turn for advice when confronted by a "grey" ethical challenge. What is your advice?

CS-M: Every wellness practitioner should be involved in individual or peer supervision! But peers also need to include trained psychotherapists. Sometimes practitioners believe they are in a grey area when they're not—it's a legal or moral issue. For example, take the whole question of pro bono work. I personally feel it's important to work with anyone who needs work, even if they can't pay for it. It's not unethical to give services freely. But you can be smart or stupid about this. Give sessions to people you care about or those who can send you new clients. My motto is this: "Do what you love and the money will come!"

Q: Many a practitioner, out of kindness, has unwittingly become embroiled in a battleground involving a warring couple, both of whom are patients, or warring directors in a local corporation or association. Do you advise the practitioner to refer one/or both of the patients to a colleague the moment details of the war situation crop up in discussions during the therapy?

CS-M: Absolutely! If the practitioner was keeping good boundaries and upholding confidentiality, these types of situations would be nipped in the bud. The problem is that if there's a history of loose boundaries, then it's difficult to avoid these types of situations. Whenever you work with people who are in relationships with other clients you need to set firm boundaries from day one. Tell each client that you totally uphold confidentiality and that means that neither party can ask you anything about what happens in the other's session—not even well-meaning inquiries such as, "Did Susie's headache abate?"

It's very important for therapists when working on two people related in any way to set very stringent boundaries from the get-go. If you work on a couple and they suddenly announce they are going through a divorce, it may be unethical/or a betrayal to refuse one or other partner treatments if you have been working on both of them for some time. How do you make a choice? You could refer both to different colleagues. It depends on the progress you have made, and what you are working on. Now this can be much more difficult if it's a battleground between doctors working on the couple in a clinic setting. It's always very important to discuss boundaries and issues with patients and achieve agreements based on their best interests.

Q: Is it ethical for a practitioner to insist on payment up front for, say, a package of 10 sessions, and/or to insist on a minimum of 10 sessions for the treatments to be effective? And if a patient is uncomfortable with the arrangement, should he/or she take advice from the Better Business Bureau or the practitioner's professional association?

CS-M: I don't think this an ethics matter at all. If a practitioner chooses to do business this way then the client has the option to go elsewhere. If the practitioner does require prepayment (which is not necessarily wise unless s/he is also giving a discount for prepayment), there should also be clear refund terms—the client might not want to continue or gets the desired results in a shorter time. The arrangement only becomes unethical when there is no recourse.

Q: Practitioner "A" discovered that her patient—who she was treating for addiction—had been receiving regular supplies of street drugs from practitioner "B" in a different field of Bodywork. Should practitioner "A" report practitioner "B" to his professional association, or should practitioner "A" advise the patient to report practitioner "B"?

CS-M: Some associations' Codes of Ethics require you to be a "snitch". But the patient—not the therapist—should be encouraged to report the practitioner, anonymously if necessary

Q: A sad case came up recently of a young Asian teenager who walked into an Acupuncture clinic desperate for an abortion because she was terrified her father would kill her. Alas in real life, the Acupuncturist

just turned her away. How would you advise any Acupuncturist or Bodyworker confronting a similar situation?

CS-M: This is a problem between what is legal, and what is ethical. The teenager was probably hoping the Acupuncturist would supply her with the necessary herbs and treatment to prompt an abortion, as she may have heard about such services in her birth country, and be unaware where she should turn for help in the USA. I'd be inclined to walk her over to Planned Parenthood for advice. I wouldn't have just turned her away.

Q: How do you advise a young practitioner re extremely needy patients who cling and became demanding and even hostile if the practitioner limits calls or refers the patient to a colleague?

CS-M: Again, if the practitioner sets healthy boundaries up front, this won't happen "as much". It's important to remember that our mission in life isn't always what it appears. The actual treatment you do might not be the key in the healing for this patient. But this kind of adulation can be annoying. It clouds the therapeutic dynamic. Maybe it's projection. Perhaps coaching such patients to be more self-reliant is the most important "medicine" that the practitioner can provide. The practitioner may need to refer the client with tact and diplomacy, explaining that the referral is to a colleague with some appropriate specialization.

Q: Sometimes practitioners overwhelm patients with procedures that don't honor a patient's request, for example, insisting a patient needs multiple needling in an Acupuncture session even if the patient requests a minimum of needles. How do you help students avoid such situations in a clinical setting?

CS-M: By reassuring them that the best treatment is not always the quickest, but the treatment the patient can handle. Practitioners who insist on certain procedures run the risk of being unethical because it's not in the patient's best interests, and because of the power differential. Given the dynamics of the situation, with a patient lying on a floor or table, with the therapist standing above them, the potential for abuse is there. People don't understand the prevalence of abuse. In practice at least a third of all patients have been abused in some way, and practitioners need to be aware of this and to respect it. Such subtleties are sometimes overlooked by therapists who have been in practice for a long time, and that's dangerous. They forget to go slowly ...

19

Building an Acupuncture Practice From Storefronts to Web Sites

KAREN E. NUNLEY, LAc, MSOM *created The Healing Acupuncture Center out of a storefront on a busy Austin street in an office plaza sandwiched between a Barbershop and a stationery store in 1996. She is a member of the board of governors of the Academy of Oriental Medicine at Austin (AOMA) and a guest teacher in the Academy's business practice management classes. She is a consultant to the Texas State Board of Acupuncture Examiners and a past member of the Board of Directors for the Texas Association of Acupuncture and Oriental Medicine. Karen volunteers with Hospice Austin using Acupuncture to provide palliative and end-of-life care. She also worked closely with AOMA and the People's Community Clinic to create a weekly student clinic that offers free Acupuncture to low income and uninsured families in Austin.*

Q: Did you create your practice out of a storefront to attract walk-in clients who may not otherwise have sought your service? We hear some of your first clients were truck drivers who saw your sign and walked in because they had back pain!

KN: I like having a storefront! I chose this space because my favorite complementary healthcare practitioner, a Chiropractor, had been in the same spot before and had just moved out. I had always liked it and have been here ever since I started my practice in 1996. For me this is better than being shut away down a hall on the second floor of a commercial building. In the beginning I had a lot of folks walk in from the barbershop next door—they saw my sign and came in. Today we still do have walk-ins but most of my new business is from word of mouth referrals and from visitors to my Web site.

Q: What are the hardest lessons you've learned in your 10 years of clinical practice about creating your own business? And do you share these details with students in your business classes?

KN: I tell the students the one of my biggest mistakes was thinking I could do it all without any help. I soon learned that giving treatments is only one of the many tasks involved in running an Acupuncture practice. When I wasn't interacting directly with patients, I needed to take care of bookkeeping, marketing, networking, inventory, housekeeping, laundry, correspondence, and even decorating. As my practice grew, so did the amount of time it took to get all these jobs done. Eight years passed when one day it hit me how smart it would be to have an advisory board that I could turn to for help and expertise in growing my practice. So I asked an MD, RN, Chiropractor, accountant and top marketing specialist if they would be willing to be on my advisory board. To my delight they all said yes!

Q: And how did they help you?

KN: My number one goal for that first gathering was to brainstorm how to keep the *flow* of my practice steadier. It had always been unpredictable, varying from overwhelmingly busy to almost non-existent. My new advisory board quickly figured it out and taught me something that was very important. When I wasn't giving a treatment, I was not generating income. Period. When I was busy, I spent the majority of my time giving treatments. I would budget little or no time on marketing and keeping the pipeline full, which resulted in the inevitable slow times. After focusing on marketing and drumming up more business, I would get very busy for a while. Then the cycle would repeat.

My advisory board unanimously agreed it was time for me to hire an office manager to run and market the business while I stayed in the treatment rooms creating income. I resisted because I didn't think I could afford to pay for help during the lean times. My board advised me to raise my rates by $10 per patient and to find a "mature" person who was retired, flexible, with a lot of professional experience and who would treat my patients as well as I did. So I followed their advice. The very next week I hired an office manager with marketing and accounting experience who works for me thirty hours a week. Now I do what I love best, working with patients, while she handles the rest. She has been a Godsend! And the flow has remained steady since she began.

Q: *In what other ways does your office manager help you?*

KN: She keeps the pipeline full by marketing on an ongoing basis to our core group. We have found that 20% of our patients are 80% of our business, split about 60:40 women to men, and so this is our target market. She e-mails studies to them which highlight the benefits of Asian Medicine for specific problems. She continually updates our Web site to keep it current and interesting. She makes phone calls the day before appointments to remind people, a nice, professional touch for which we get positive feedback. She welcomes patients as they come in, and answers their phone calls promptly. Patients feel cared for from the first moment. She handwrites thank you notes to everyone who sends us a referral. We do not give discounts to patients in exchange for referrals—we find that they refer us because they value our service.

Q: *How have you refined your marketing planning so you can balance the fruitful months with the skinny months?*

KN: My very first year in practice, I bought two hours of time from a healthcare marketing consultant who gave me great advice: "Unlike medical doctors in the insurance world, you will not be receiving referrals, so you will need to build your practice through networking and shaking hands. Don't waste money on newspaper advertising or buying expensive space in the yellow pages. Get out there, meet people one on one, and hand out your business cards."

With Austin's numerous high tech companies, I was able to participate in many health fairs right after getting my license. I ran a beautiful booth with professional handouts, met a lot of people and handed out hundreds of business cards and brochures. I also volunteered to give talks about Asian Medicine in offices and at networking meetings. I knew that even if I just picked up a few new clients per event, they would usually refer one to five more to me by word of mouth.

Meeting people one on one has been the main source of business for me over the last ten years. I always carry business cards with me—even to the grocery store!

Q: What other recommendations do you offer your students?

KN: I recommend that new practitioners create a network of other talented specialists they can refer to and receive referrals from, like Chiropractors, Massage Therapists, Asian Bodywork Therapists, Psychotherapists and MDs. You can offer a trade or go to the practitioner as a patient. If you like their work and style, you can discuss establishing a mutually beneficial referral relationship with them. We keep a box of business cards on hand of all the practitioners we refer. Being able to recommend a good referral is an important service for our patients and they really appreciate it.

Q: How do you advise your students to attract patients based on your own experience?

KN: I have learned that according to the universal law of attraction, life is much easier when we focus on what we want rather than what we don't want, and let go of worrying about the "how" of making it happen. So I try to focus on attracting the kind of patients I would most like to serve, and have crafted a list of the exact characteristics of my "perfect/ideal patient", as: joyful, fun, spiritual, high integrity, heart-centered, open-minded, loyal, committed to his/his own healing, and able to communicate health-related needs, compliant, and gladly refers at least one new like-minded patient to us monthly, and happily pays our fee. I like to read and tweak this ever-evolving list as often as every day because we attract those on whom we focus. I have found that it has made a *huge* difference in the quality of our patients. The majority of them are such a joy to work with, and I truly love going to work every day.

Q: We hear that some students roll their eyes when you give them advice. Do they think starting a practice is just a matter of hanging up a shingle?

KN: That is certainly what I thought when I first started. I have made my fair share of mistakes and have learned a lot. Now I search for as many ideas as I can on how to be successful in my practice. I think some graduates may not really be ready to practice full-time. Most are so fried toward the end of their training and can only focus on getting out of school and passing their exams. They are not ready to think about the challenges of starting a business!

Q: How do you teach students to promote their specializations?

KN: I explain that they need to be sensitive to what the market is seeking. For example, if students are going to practice in Austin, they need to be good at treating allergies and pain, as that is why many people seek Acupuncture. Other people are waiting longer to begin families, so fertility is becoming a timely condition for Acupuncture treatment. I also have a lot of baby boomers coming in for cosmetic Acupuncture. New practitioners need to pay attention to trends and stay up-to-date on Continuing Education.

Q: What do you think of the idea of using Web sites, blogs, and internet chat rooms as a way of expanding a practice?

KN: Our Web site, which has been a big plus for the business, attracts at least two new patients a week. Most of their preliminary questions are answered by the FAQs on the Web site, so when they call us they are ready to schedule. I highly recommend a thorough and informative website as a way of expanding a practice.

To consider spending time answering blog and internet questions, I would have to hire more staff to help me.

Q: What inspired you to help create an offsite student clinic at Austin's People's Community Clinic?

KN: It is so important to give back to the community. I wanted to create a situation where I could go and give Acupuncture to those who could not afford it, but I didn't want the administrative headache of setting up and running a free Acupuncture clinic. I wanted somebody else to schedule the appointments, run the space, so I could just show up and be more hands-on with the patients. At the same time AOMA was looking for an opportunity to create a student clinic in a community setting. The two ideas came together and merged, resulting in the creation of the fist Acupuncture student clinic in a conventional healthcare setting in Austin.

Q: Do you believe students should complete internships at community clinics or in organizations like Acupuncture Without Borders?

KN: I think it's an excellent idea. I would also like to see more student clinics in hospice, pediatric clinics, and of course, in hospitals as well.

D: ECLECTIC METHODOLOGY

.... Hence the Zen search for other and better ways to convey experience. These methods, a shout, a blow, a paradox of gesture, silence itself, are more direct as a medium.—Christmas Humphreys—*Zen Buddhism (1)*

Scholars call Socrates' method the elenchus, *which is Hellenistic Greek for inquiry or cross-examination. But it is not just any type of inquiry or examination. It is a type that reveals people to themselves.*—Christopher Phillips—*Socrates Café (2)*

WANDERING calligraphy by Yuxia Qiu, LAc

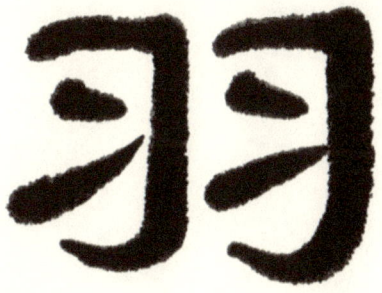

20

The Alchemy and Art of the Demonstration

LINDY FERRIGNO, Dipl ABT (NCCAOM), AOBTA®-CI, LMT *has played a major role in the development of Shiatsu training since 1977 in schools, community colleges and Acupuncture colleges from the east to the west coast in the United States, and in schools in Germany. She was one of a dozen people across the U.S. who spearheaded the founding of the AOBTA, and a team player in the development of national exams and standards in Asian Bodywork Therapy. Her unique practice in Charlottesville Virginia also reflects her years of advanced studies in Shiatsu with Pauline Sasaki and Shinmei Kishi, her studies with American and French Osteopaths, and with a Cherokee elder. She mainly teaches Continuing Education now as she enjoys the freedom to lead people beyond the rudimentary knowledge base to the art of healing.*

Q: *What is your best teaching method for demonstrating meridians? Do you teach a Yin/Yang pair on the same day so students can feel the different qualities of Yin and Yang? Do you get the students to track meridians on their own bodies first, with stretches, and movement, before you demonstrate the meridian location and dynamic on the model?*

LF: I teach the students Yin and Yang in pairs but not so that they can feel the different qualities back to back. I do it to give some sense of order to the system. I like to teach the meridian as a whole first, otherwise students get hung up on the points and I want them to feel the meridian and the body as a whole. This makes it easier for the students to grasp. This blends more easily with theory, too, when you teach the five element associations. I ask students to refer to their text and trace the meridians on themselves prior to the class. If they come in prepared they will have a good idea of the general location of those meridians. They pair up in class and I go around and help them precisely locate the meridians. Once they are actually *on* the meridians, they can feel the different qualities much more easily. I teach the traditional meridians first to familiarize students with the common TCM locations. Then I teach Shizuto Masunaga's extended meridians and emphasize the expanded meridian system throughout the course.

Q: What is your art of teaching acupoints to enable students to locate and feel the quality of the different energetics of each point? Do you teach points as you teach the appropriate meridian? Or later?

LF: I teach the meridians first and then go back and teach the points so the students don't get hung up on each point. I do not teach the energetics of each point. Instead, I teach the function of the meridian in a million different ways and in a million different words because that information forms an important part of the foundations of Zen Shiatsu, which is my base.

Q: What do you most enjoy demonstrating?

LF: Treatment of pathologies! Within a classroom, for instance, you've gone through x, y and z meridians, now you have a pathology such as temporal headaches, involving Gall Bladder and Triple Warmer meridians. I take what they have learned and put it into the context of a treatment to show how it works. The theory augments the treatment rather than the treatment augmenting the theory. I make believe that someone has the symptoms if there is nobody in the class who actually has them. Students see that there is more than a technique to what we are doing. I speak aloud while I demonstrate the treatment, tell them what my thinking is, tell them what I feel, and how I put it all together. This adds dimension, but really it is the hardest piece of the work and it is the heart of the work. Students often don't realize how much they have to change themselves to work the alchemy of healing.

Q: Could you share your thoughts on the "alchemy" of healing?

LF: The way I see it, part of our work as teachers and Bodyworkers is to perform this normal human activity at a higher level. We transform the *science* of teaching into the *art* of teaching, or the *art* of healing. That is why I use the word "alchemy." Its original meaning refers to the endeavor to manifest the spiritual mystery at the heart of the material universe. It is the effort to infuse the physical body with the energy of Creation Source. Alchemy happens when you believe in the magic and beauty that is life, when you see the reality of it all around and act on the knowledge that the laws of the universe support this phenomenon.

Q: Could you give us an example from your classroom?

LF: Toward the end of one class a student mentioned that her thumb had been swollen for several years following an accident, and that no treatment had been able to provide lasting relief. I asked her if she would be open to a group healing by the class and she agreed. I told the class to stay in touch with the goal of facilitating the healing, and to be aware of how much energy they were putting out, both individually and collectively. It's important not to over-stimulate. Some classmates did Shiatsu on the student. Others provided healing energy by placing their hands on those who gave Shiatsu. Their desire to help their classmate was almost palpable. They paid attention. No one did too much and everyone experienced the end of the treatment at the same moment. They gently removed their hands, one by one, and sat quietly for a moment. Everyone had been deeply moved. Then we looked at her hand. All the swelling was gone and she cried tears of gratitude. I knew the student for another two years, and the swelling never returned during that time.

This was a clear case of everyone involved in transforming him/herself, and the room, into a healing space for the student/client. Their desire to help, their concentration of love, and their belief in what they were doing brought about the right conditions for healing to occur. They called this forth from what they had inside themselves and made it special for that situation. It was so beautiful.

Q: How do you organize your demonstrations? If you have to demo a particular sequence of techniques, do you show students the entire sequence first, then break the sequence into a logical order of "building blocks", giving students a chance to practice each block first before linking the blocks together?

LF: No, I do just the opposite. I show pieces first and then put it together, kind of like the way I learned to ballroom dance—you learn this step then you learn that step and then you put it all together to dance.

Q: What is your advice for working with students who have dyslexia or similar learning challenges?

LF: I don't necessarily consider people as learning disabled, because I think many people who are attracted to our hands-on profession have a different way of learning. Instead of spending a lot of time explaining a particular technique during a demonstration, I tell them not to worry if they don't grasp it because when we get to practicing I will help them personally. This is more personal, they're not worried, and when they don't worry they can take in the learning kinesthetically through touch.

Q: Some students learn techniques very quickly; others take a long time and need frequent guidance. Do you encourage fast and slow lanes to work together?

LF: I have found that fast and slow people working together agitate each other. They don't get the kind of feedback that they need. If the slow person goes first, the fast person going second does not get the time they need to practice the session. If I notice this dynamic, I give warnings, so I give them x amount of time, then warn them that they are half way through, five minutes left, then one minute left, then time to switch. If you are running behind, don't speed up I tell them. Just leave something out.

Q: List some of the worst—and some of the most inspirational—demonstrations you have observed?

LF: The worst example happens when the teacher doesn't notice that the demonstration is making the model feel uncomfortable—either emotionally or physically. If the teacher can't turn the situation around and make it ok for the model and the class, it's a bad demo. It's also bad when the teacher can't talk and work at the same time, or when the teacher starts a sentence and drops it. However, at times there is value to a teacher saying "I am going to demonstrate without talking, please hold your questions until the end." This shows students the order, rhythm and meditative attention that goes into treatment.

What most inspired me as a student and informed my teaching style, was when the instructor was not just demonstrating the technique, but caused a change in the model, and the students could see and feel the change. It is the way you concentrate and set your intention that makes miracles possible. I like to set up the demonstration to wow the students. I want them to be awed by the power and beauty of this thing that we do—and I want to encourage them to go for *that*.

Q: A common mistake among many teachers is to overload theory and then cram the demo and practice time into the last hour of class. How do you time your demonstrations—before or after a lot of theory?

LF: I like one third of theory and demo, and two thirds of student practice and Q&A. I like students to do a routine before asking questions and then ask more questions at the end; I like their questions to come directly from their experiences.

Q: What recommendations do you have for a teacher who wishes to perfect the art of practical demonstrations? What techniques or information sources have you incorporated as you developed your own expertise?

LF: I recommend that they rehearse: demonstrate in front of a mirror, time themselves, and practice talking simultaneously while demonstrating. Do dress rehearsals with an audience of non-bodyworkers. If people don't know the subject matter they can easily identify for you what is clear and what isn't.

I don't enjoy watching teachers just for sheer technique. I like people who transform things. I have apprenticed with Zen Shiatsu instructors, Osteopaths, Chiropractors, and have studied for many years under indigenous healers, Celtic, Cherokee and Shinto. I incorporate what I've learned from the personage of each teacher, not only their techniques. This is why I recommend self-development. Development of expertise comes from many factors, your own experience, knowledge, and intuitive knowing. When teaching, intuition means staying in touch with your purpose and sensing whether or not your students are getting it. Creating an atmosphere of respect and protection for your students allows them to do their own healing and develop their gifts. It's all about using you own *Qi* to transform the atmosphere in the classroom.

Q: How do you select models for your demonstrations? Do you provide any direction to models prior to working on them or during a demonstration?

LF: I let people volunteer. Now and then I ask, "Who has not been demonstrated on yet?" Or, I will ask a person at the back of the class who is chatting and not paying attention, to come forward to be a model. This removes distraction and restores function to the classroom. Before each class I arrange my *Qi* to make my classroom conducive to learning. I verbally set up boundaries for confidentiality at the very beginning of a course. I let people go through a range of feelings, let things happen even if people have to face their own issues. If I sense a very delicate situation, then I will not push. I let people break down a little bit or get belligerent and allow them to work through their stuff. However, that is only because I am trained by indigenous healers to help people through these issues. I take this responsibility very seriously. I want to help them "healer, heal thyself."

Q: What is the best way to manage a class of multiple students and models practicing on each other? For example, do you move among the groups, or do you observe from one point and approach a group only when called upon?

LF: I do both things. I move among the groups when I have just taught something new. I critique with encouraging feedback like "don't be afraid, go ahead and try …" as well as making corrections in posture and technique. But during a 12 week course, you review things many times, so sometimes the students need a chance to practice without interrupting their flow. In these instances, I will not do anything unless I see they may harm themselves or their partner or if they call me over. I take notes and give written feedback to the students so they know what they need to work on and what they are doing well. Personally, I prefer to know what I am doing wrong so it took me a while to realize that people need positive reinforcement, too. It helps them know what strengths they can build on.

Q: What advice do you give students to help them work with patients who are dying?

LF: I tell them that they themselves have to be comfortable with the death process. If they are not comfortable they should seek therapy or spiritual counseling to come to a place of peace about it. Also the practitioner's ideas and beliefs may have no relevance to the way a person deals with his/her own death. They must deal with a patient on the patient's terms, according to his/her physical and emotional comfort levels.

For instance, I had a patient who first came to me in the final stages of liver cancer. He looked emaciated and it scared me. But I did the best I could. Shiatsu gave him a lot of pain relief so that he could sleep through the night. He came every week until he died three months later. During that time his wife confided in me that she was concerned he was not facing the fact that he was dying. He would not talk about it with her, wouldn't even let her bring up the subject of his father's death a few months previously. But he *would* speak to me about his father, even though he would not allow any talk of his own impending death. However, it was clear to me, through responses of his energetic field, that he was aware of his time and that he was dealing with it privately.

Practitioners have to respect that and let patients do it their own way. And it is best to give dying patients short sessions with a light touch, so you don't deplete energy. And don't be overtly sentimental; you need to be clear, calm and helpful. Even when you do all this, working with the dying can get to you, as it did with me when a large number of patients died in a short span of time when I was working in an AIDS clinic. You must do your own self care, get rest, and get treatments. And, talk to other people who have been there, and will understand this particular, profound type of grief experienced by hospice workers and caretakers of the dying.

21

The Value of Dojo Training in Asian Medicine

JEFFREY DANN, PhD, LAc, AOBTA®-CI *is a medical anthropologist who researched his master's thesis on the streets of Seattle to study patterns of drinking and socialization among urbanized Native Americans. This prompted him to seek a more holistic approach which he found within the Asian martial arts and healing arts of Japan. His intensive Dojo training included Kendo (yondan), iadi-do (nidan), naginata-do (shodan) at Mito Tobukan Dojo in Ibaraki Prefecture. His Dojo education in Japanese manual medicine was in Seitai Jutsu (corrective exercise) and Shiatsu under sensei Miyata Tomei, kendo kyoshi nanadan. After studying Acupuncture in Hong Kong, China, Hawaii, and Japan he created the Traditional Japanese Acupuncture Foundation of Hawaii in 1984 with sensei Chieko Maekawa. He lives in Colorado where he runs the Aloha Wellness Clinic in Boulder. His teaching combines structural approaches of Japanese manual medicine systems.*

Q: You've emphasized the importance of Dojo training in Japanese life as going way beyond training in the martial arts or the western zeal for "going to the gym". Can you summarize the Dojo value for you as a western student of Japanese martial arts and Japanese Medicine?

JD: *Katei kyoiku* or family education is the teaching of values of the home among family members, the nucleus of deep family relationships and support. *Gakko kyoiku* or school education is for building successive layers of knowledge to be an informed intelligent contributing member of society. *Dojo kyoiku* or Dojo education is the place where they learn mutual respect and mindfulness in the context of effort and struggle with peers.

Dojo education has a value for the academic training of Asian Medicine because it provides a valuable container for mindfulness, respect, and concentration in the sometimes disruptive competitive arena of the school environment. Cleanliness, mental preparation, humility, mutual respect, co-ordination of body-mind, and spirit are valuable additions to the learning environment.

Q: Is Dojo training fundamental to your work with students?

JD: I do try to bring a unification of intent and mindfulness into the opening of my classes in Acupuncture and Bodywork programs. This might include Qigong, movement, breathwork, and brief meditation.

I include many Dojo rules. For example, shoes are lined up inside the door, and I discourage eating during the class or other forms of personal distraction. It's good to have an opening and closing that focuses mind, body, and spirit, like the *rei* (bow) in the Dojo, or breath, or even toning.

Q: Ideally what comes first, training in Kendo or Aikido to lay the groundwork for a future training in Traditional Japanese Medicine, or should the training be concurrent?

JD: I think that a concurrent Dojo education approach for beginning Acupuncture students would be ideal. It is perhaps the only way that beginning students can begin to *embody* many of the principles and teachings which otherwise would remain only in their heads. But because training in a *budo* (martial art) is a long term commitment, I feel that softer, more internal, reflective forms like Tai Chi or Qigong are more valuable in the healing arts than external, explosive forms like Aikido or Kendo.

Soft inner movement forms can teach a beginner more effectively in a limited time in more focused body-mind-spirit consciousness, rather than a highly developed martial body-mind skill set.

Q: Do any of your American students resist the practical aspects of Dojo training like the ritual cleaning of the Dojo floor, opening and closing the Dojo? How do you convince them that this is all part of

essential Ki training, in terms of how they move, and how they prepare Ki space for themselves and for the group?

JD: Yes, this is a big problem for some students who perceive Dojo education as a demeaning form of abuse by a school or teacher. They might feel that since they are paying tuition to gain a career that they shouldn't have to sweep the floors, observe behaviors that support a sacred ceremonial space in which to learn.

It is important to acknowledge and address the special issues of Body-Mind learning and the value of creating a special environment to cultivate those qualities of the Asian culture and mind that embrace everything the student has come to learn. I introduce some basic fundamentals of meditation, breathing, and Qigong movements to clear, settle, and generate *Ki*. I introduce experiential exercises to help students embody principles of *Ki*, movement, and feeling within Asian Medicine. If they don't see the learning environment as a special and sacred place then they shouldn't be in my program.

Q: What are the major differences you have discovered between Chinese and Japanese Medicine?

JD: The Chinese love symmetrically ordered richly complex interwoven details of relationship (this is mirrored in the extremely fine breakdown of TCM differential diagnosis) while the Japanese appreciate the more fundamental aspects of the elegance of asymmetrical simplicity. And Japanese Medicine loves the concept of simultaneous diagnosis and treatment. The Japanese approach seems to look-palpate for re-confirmation as the session progresses. Does the pulse change? Does the abdomen relax? Do the hard areas soften? Does the structure shift? If not, the treatment plan needs to change.

Q: How do you share your structural alignment techniques (Balancing the Koshi and Sotai Ho) with your students? As many of the techniques require detailed awareness of Anatomy and Physiology, and the patient's history, how do you prepare your students to modify or minimize specific techniques? I am thinking specifically of the technique where, in prone position, you slide the patient's knee up as high as possible and then straighten the patient's leg in a single sharp

movement. This would be impossible on anyone with knee problems, or a senior citizen, or anyone with a chronic pelvic imbalance.

JD: At the core of my teaching is the dictum that if it hurts, don't do it. Only go to the stage of "that feels like a good hurt." Practitioners must get a clear history of injury or disability and advise the patient to speak up if any procedure is painful or even prompts a fear of pain.

If the practitioner is taught to listen in palpation before and during a movement, any restrictions can be noted and nothing is forced beyond a physiological or emotional limit.

Of course knowledge of Anatomy and Physiology is fundamental both for Bodywork and for Acupuncture students. For severe limitations of injury, disability, or age, I teach students how to modify or even eliminate certain moves. For these situations the ability to know when and how to switch from the *Sei Tai* passive mobilizations that work at the limits of the range of motion to a more gentle limited *Sotai* active Range-of-Motion is important, and valuable.

Q: Your Koshi workshops emphasized the idiomatic use of "Koshi" in the Japanese language to imply aspects of torso and postural alignment/ distortion (like koshi ga suwaru—to be grounded) and you also used terms like "Tensegrity" from Buckminster Fuller's "dome" designs, to emphasize the importance of achieving harmonious movement and function through structural alignment. Do you also integrate this imagery into group meditations with your students so they can visualize the associations in internal Ki exercises before they start to practice the Koshi?

JD: I think I'm more interested in having students *feel* the body-mind of these concepts than to *imagine* them. Experiential anatomy gives me more mileage then initial imagining. I prefer *imaging* for exploring the internal landscape of the viscera, meridians, and elements.

Q: You also highlighted the importance of the Gall Bladder meridian, in terms of location and key points (like GB 41, 29, 30), as major players for structural alignment. Could you share a case study from your own clinical practice to illustrate your Koshi applications (either in rehab, or to treat, say, a Sacro-Iliac twist?)

JD: Let's take the case of the "Colorado Cowboy" in the mountain town of La Veta, Southern Colorado. Young men raised in this region often entered youth, county and state rodeo events—hard working country men, stoic and tough. "Colorado Cowboy", a 42 year old former state brahma bull riding champ, had become a broken down rancher on workman's comp disability. He could barely bend over to take off his boots. This 6'2" 300 lb rancher's *Koshi* was severely pulled forward and distorted on the left side. His Gall Bladder meridian was "corkscrewed", compressed at the Tensor Fascia Lata, especially around GB 29 which aggravated his lumbar lordosis and compressed his left sacro-iliac joint. After three treatments, his *Koshi* distortion was significantly balanced to the extent that he had dramatic relief from pain. His movement improved so much he was able to return to work on his ranch. The key to releasing his left posterior lumbar sacro-iliac pain and dysfunction was to unwind the front of the pelvic Dai Mai belt meridian.

Q: What specific techniques of Sotai Ho and Koshi have you found to be the most clinically useful, combined with Shiatsu and Japanese Acupuncture? And do you perform these techniques before or after needling?

JD: Japanese manual systems have dual aspects, a spectrum of touch and movement that may be used for assessment as well as for active treatment. So I tend to use my hands first in assessment and sometimes that leads into immediate *Sotai-Seitai*-Shiatsu moves. At other times, these manual assessments lead to Acupuncture first. We move between structure and energy, between structure and function. More often, balancing the pulse is done more powerfully and quickly with Acupuncture (Treating the Root), and then manual therapies might follow to address structural limitations.

Q: What do you emphasize in your training courses in Japanese-style Acupuncture for MDs in Turkey?

JD: In Turkey, only MD's can practice Acupuncture. This presents a certain difficulty because of the pre-existing Western allopathic mindset. They are still conditioned, first of all, to get a western disease name and then ask for a formulary of points to treat that Western disease. They don't understand at first the issue of grasping the underlying pattern of imbalance. Also, they tend to appreciate electro-diagnostic machinery that finds and treats points, machines that buzz and beep and have active screens. This means like most Western Medical doctors, they don't trust their hands for palpatory diagnosis and tend not to do pulse, abdominal, or meridian diagnosis. And as with many western physicians they rely on Western diagnostics. My basic goals in Turkey have been to introduce the fundamentals of Japanese Meridian therapy, to teach palpatory skills to assess underlying deficiency, and to needle gently, superficially, and appropriately for deficient root patterns. Also, to recheck both pulse and local sites of deficiency or excess with reconfirmation during and after treatment.

Many of the MDs already using Acupuncture or who want to use it, are anesthesiologists, rather than MDs in physical medicine or rehab. But recently I taught a bunch of dentists—interestingly—all women—some of whom had spent time in Japan, and realized that their own dentistry training was too narrow. They sought a more wholistic approach because they knew there was so much in the jaw and face related to the emotions. Similarly they wanted to know more about structural/emotional issues related to the cervical spine.... whereas the anesthesiologists are often just looking for pain management.

22

Exploring Pulse Diagnosis

WILLIAM MORRIS, DAOM, MSEd, LAc *is president of the Academy of Oriental Medicine at Austin, Texas, and president emeritus of the American Association of Acupuncture and Oriental Medicine (AAAOM)*

Q: Everyone tells us you have a very special way of teaching pulse diagnosis. Can you share some of your experiences?

WM: I use pulse diagnosis as a monitor for treatment. It is a microcosm of the whole person. In a holographic sense, the pulse reflects the structures and processes of the individual in their environment.

My first experiences with pulse diagnosis were based upon *shape* and *volume.* This method often provides a simple and clear set of observations. I worked this way for years prior to learning about the twenty-seven basic pulse qualities.

Because of the confidence these early practices gave me, I focus on shape and volume first when teaching others. The complexities of vessel tension, force, turbulence and the wave come later. This creates a sense of confidence which is vital…. Trust what you feel.

I use metaphors, graphic demonstrations drawings and available objects to convey the images. Most important is to sit with the learner and identify pulses in real time.

Teaching the pulse requires first description, then demonstration, and lastly, guided practice. Some teachers bring rubber tubing into the classroom to demonstrate different shapes, bulging in one area or small in another area. Sometimes I will use string or wire to demonstrate the tension of a wiry pulse—here, the nervous system causes the vascular system to tighten when the person is stressed.

Demonstration of a slippery pulse is performed by sliding my finger nails quickly past the tips of the student's fingers. I then find a student with a very slippery pulse and have the other students palpate.

Q: *What other methods do you use to demonstrate pulses?*

WM: Part of what creates a powerful learning experience, is the ability of the teacher to break the process down into discrete pieces. The practitioner focuses on one piece of data collection at a time. This helps to disarm the assumption that pulse diagnosis is difficult. It is essential to have demonstration with guided practice. Ideally, a senior practitioner helps a student in the classroom and then in supervised clinic.

The use of western physiological, anatomical and physics models may also assist the pulse student in the process of grasping the pulse. There is a pump, fluid, tubes and ground substance where the tubes rest.

We know that senior learners grow and learn effectively through teaching. The best students get sufficient repetition of the material in the order of 100–200 hours. When they began to teach modules of the work or even full seminars; a whole new level of learning occurs.

Q: *Can pulse Qi change during verbal interaction?*

WM: Yes, the pulse changes under a variety of circumstances. If pulse is taken during dialogue, it will respond to various issues as they arise. It is an eye-opening experience for students to see how pulses shift during clinical interactions.

Different diagnostics may have variable findings, and it is important to understand why. Differences in technique can cause low inter-rater reliability. It is up to all parties to understand the reasons they are not making the same observation. The most common problem is variance in position and depth of pressure. Here is an example of technique as a cause for inconsistent findings—if I press the surface of the vessel, I am more likely to feel the surface tension of the vessel. If you press into the blood stream, however, you are likely to label the pulse as slippery if there is turbulence in the blood stream.

It can be difficult to accept this fact, the pulse changes. And these changes provide important information. There are complex physiological processes occurring, and the pulse expresses these as 'changing qualities over time.' For instance, if there is *Qi* depletion the pulse lacks force. If there is also heat and *Qi* stagnation, then the pulse can change from weak to 'wiry with some urgency.'

The pulses may also change because the *Qi* is depleted. *Qi* has 'holding' function, In this case, the pulse has trouble holding a form due to *Qi* depletion. If the *Qi* depletion is related to weak *Wei Qi* (defensive *Qi*) then the pulse can readily change in the presence of different practitioners. This last circumstance requires sensitivity on the part of the practitioner, especially if they have strong *Qi* which can be overpowering.

It is important to consider features that change and those that do not. A deep or weak pulse can change, but hardened arterial walls will not. Often a deep pulse reflects a retreat of the psyche. If psychosocial factors cause a deep pulse, it will often change with interaction. Substantial pathogens however, are less likely to change. If the pulse is substantially slippery, it won't change, it tends to be robust. A man with a full and pounding pulse won't tend to weaken. But a changing pulse is something to describe—it may cycle through wiry to weak to slippery requiring us to record the changes over time, as each cycle expresses a different pathology.

Q: Do you believe students should have the same teacher for pulse?

WM: No. However, at first, it is important to have consistency. Later, it is important to be exposed to various perspectives. I always try to have teaching assistants with me so students get both aspects.

Q: How do you teach your students to recognize a patient's substance abuse habits through pulse diagnosis?

WM: Cocaine impacts the cardiovascular and nervous systems. A person may have a hard wiry pulse by their mid twenties if they abuse during their teens. This is an age inappropriate pulse condition. And that's what we look for. With alcoholism, if the liver becomes cirrhotic, the left middle position tends to feel harder and wire like.

Q: Can you feel the damaging effect cocaine has on the San Jiao, in pulse diagnosis?

WM: It depends on the pulse method used. Cocaine can cause a breakdown in communication between the middle, upper and lower burners. Compare the distal, middle and proximal positions with each other in order to understand the way that they communicate. One can also palpate the superficial aspect of the right proximal position. The pulse will initially become more urgent and then more weak, eventually the vessel gets harder under the influence of cocaine.

With marijuana users, the left middle position lacks root, it floats. The physiological explanation for this is that marijuana causes glycogen dumping from the liver. Over time, this depletes the *Qi* of the liver and the root diminishes.

Q: Do interpretations of pulses shift from one era to the next?

WM: Yes—in fact some pulse images have fallen out of favor such as those related to the eight extraordinary vessels. I am happy to say however, that this method is making a return in the west. My doctoral dissertation explored the interpretation of distortions in the radial pulse. It explored Han Dynasty (100CE) texts such as the *Mai Jing Chapter Ten,* (3) and the *Nei Jing Chapter Four* (2). Another interpretation came from the famous Shanghai Ding family lineage, which I learned it from Shen and Hammer during the 1990s (Scheid, 2007; B. Wang, 1997a; S. Wang, 1997b) (see refs:1, 2, 3). These easily identified pulse shapes are not in the mainstream texts, yet they lead to effective clinical interventions. One has to wonder how it is that medical practices fall into and out of favor. These decisions are not based upon best practices, but they are in part, socially constructed.

Q: Many students complain that, in some schools, too much emphasis is placed on memorizing pulse qualities, rates, and rhythms, and not

enough emphasis on experience and practice in class. How do you help students develop their practical skills?

WM: Memorization of the pulse images is a basic requirement. Guided practice is also essential. Best practices require both. If the student is not capable of describing the pulse, they will certainly not be able to identify it on their own. But this is only a start. It is through demonstration and guided practice that the learners gain the necessary skills in pulse diagnosis.

The primary problem in mainstream school curricula is the amount of classroom training that is dedicated to pulse diagnosis. In most US Acupuncture and Asian Medicine programs, there are three to ten classroom hours dedicated to introductory pulse diagnosis work. These studies are followed with discussion during the internal medicine and clinical portions of the training. However, there seems to be a universal perception that there is insufficient pulse diagnosis training.

Q: Do you believe that your background in Asian Bodywork makes you that much more sensitive to the qualities of Qi, touch and subtle pressure required of pulse diagnosis?

WM: Yes. My first education in pulse diagnosis came with the Asian Bodywork training. I was trained to take the pulse in order to select that channel or points. I would then take the pulse again as a monitor for efficacy. Using the hands this way increases sensitivity.

Q: Some students find it hard to distinguish between, a choppy and an irregular pulse, or between a tight and a wiry pulse. How do you help them develop sensitivity to the differences, or do you reassure them that this comes with experience?

WM: Experience is necessary, but good instruction is also a key. However, the terms we use to describe the pulse are part of the problem. For instance, when we translate *se mai* the terms 'rough' and 'choppy pulse' are both used by different authorities. Kaptchuk (7) uses the term 'irregular pulse' as a descriptor for a choppy pulse. This refers to irregularities in rhythm. Further, arrhythmias are sometimes called irregular. The *dai mai* is usually translated as 'intermittent,' it is a regularly missed beat, possibly, every seven beats the pulse misses. The *jie mai* is usually translated as 'knotted,' it is an irregularly irregular pulse. I tell them that assurance comes with confidence in the knowledge and the descriptions and terms. Once we have felt the pulse in the clinic together and have confirmed each other's observations, confidence increases.

The tight and wiry pulses are distinguished in response to another question. However, descriptions of the choppy pulse over the millennia have been confusing. To itemize a few, **the choppy pulse ...**

- **Jin Wei:** ... is fine, slow, short, scattered, hesitant, and unsmooth, like scraping bamboo with a knife. (4)

- **Maciocia:** ... feels rough under the finger: instead of a smooth pulse wave, it feels as though it had a jagged edge to it. Choppy also indicates a pulse that changes rapidly both in rate and quality. (5)

- **Li Shizhen:** ... feels thin, minute and short and has an uneven flow, beating three and five times with an irregular rhythm. It feels like a knife scraping bamboo, rough and jagged. It is easily scattered like rain falling onto the sand. It also moves very slowly and at irregular depths, like an ill silkworm eating a leaf. (6)

- **Wang Shuhe:** ... is fine and slow, coming and going with difficulty and scattered or with an interruption. (3)

- **Kaptchuk:** ... is irregular in rhythm. In this case it is called the three and five not adjusted, sometimes three beats per breath and sometimes five beats per breath. (7)

- **Deng Tietao:** ... should feel slow and uneven, fine, small, short. (9)

- **Chinese Acupuncture and Moxibustion:** ... is a hesitant pulse that feels rough and uneven. Stagnations produce a hesitant and forceful pulse, whereas insufficiency creates a hesitant and weak pulse. (8)

There are four aspects of the pulse that can be *se*, that is, choppy or uneven. The strength or forcefulness can be uneven and changing, the frequency can be changing, or the locations and the shape can be uneven. The first question to ask is "what aspect of the pulse is uneven?"

Q: How do you help them distinguish between a tight and a wiry pulse?

WM: The *jin mai* is the tight pulse, it 'rises and falls with strength and vibrates to the left and right. It feels like fingers on a tightly stretched twisted cord.' The *xian* *mai* is the wiry pulse. It feels 'taut, long and strong, whether under pressure or not, and passes straight under the fingers. It is like a string stretched on a violin.' However, these descriptions are not enough to clarify.

The most distinguishing difference between the tight and wiry pulses is the movement side to side in the tight pulse. To feel this, place the fingers where they are touching the peak of the wave, and ask yourself this question, "does this pulse hit my fingers in the *same* spot every time?" If the answer no it is likely a tight pulse. Seek to rule out the presence of a cold pathogen when this occurs.

Lastly, the word 'vibration' as a description of the tight pulse can be confusing. In English, this implies a fairly quick motion. The movement of the crest of the wave in a tight pulse from ulna to radius can be a very slow cycle.

Q: What sort of imagery do you use to help students sense different pulses?

WM: There are many images and models. An example it the seasonal influences that are discussed in the *Spiritual Axis (B. Wang, 1997a)* (2) In spring the plants are pushing up and the pulse is wiry, reflecting the pressure it takes to emerge. In summer the plants are in full bloom and the pulse is flooding, it is full because the vessels are expanded with the heat of summer. In fall, the leaves begin to drop, the pulse becomes a little rough as the *Qi* begins to retreat and the fullness of summer is not there to support the fullness of the pulse. In the winter the pulse is deep in the presence of the influence of cold and the retreat that takes place as the days are shorter. I also use physiological descriptions. For instance a wiry pulse occurs when the nervous system causes tension in the vessel. I will also pull out a string so that the tension and linear quality of the pulse can be felt.

Q: How do you encourage your students to develop extra sensitivity in their fingertips? Do you teach them special Qi exercises for their hands and fingers?

WM: It is important to gain confidence in findings that are obvious before searching for the subtle qualities. I recommend taking as many pulses as possible under guidance. Do what it takes to make that happen. It can also be helpful to take your own pulses before and after eating as well as before and after other activities. As for the sensitivities, it is important to practice Qigong and meditation. Lastly, touch your finger tips and seek the most sensitive spot—use that for palpating.

There are physical limitations, Guitar players and people with fingers that are very large and thick skinned may not identify very subtle findings. Yet, practitioners with conical shaped fingers may have greater sensitivity. Each of these situations is a double—edged sword. Practitioners who are very sensitive can often collect so much data through the finger tips that it is difficult to sort. The larger more thick skinned fingers may not catch subtle impressions. This is OK because the obvious signs regularly drive our clinical processes.

Q: What assignments do you set your students to help them develop sensitivity to the range of pulse qualities taken at three depths and in three positions? Do you ask them to go out into the community and test dozens of different pulses?

WM: There are three steps. The first is calibration so that everyone uses the same technique and agrees as to the description and expectation. Second is guided practice. Third is practice on as many patients as possible. There is also an online pulse diagnosis support group pulsediagnosis@yahoogroups.com This allows input from an international range of practitioners.

Q: What advice do you give students who become confused over seemingly conflicting diagnostic readings between tongue and pulse?

WM: It is important to develop a tolerance for ambiguity and paradox. The basic job is to record what one observes. It is possible for many complex processes to occur simultaneously.

There is an excellent discussion about disparity between pulse and tongue findings in Tietao Deng's book, *Practical Diagnosis in Traditional Chinese Medicine* (9) in the passage on 'Precedence of the Pulse or the Signs.' When disparity of pulse and tongue occurs, the disease process is more complicated and one must sort the true from the false, this is known as the theory of 'precedence and abandoning.' If the pulse is correct and the other signs are not, abandon the signs. If the signs are correct and the pulse is not, abandon the pulse.

Q: What other advice do you give students to help simplify their pulse diagnosis?

WM: First—focus on pulse diagnostic features that you find easy. This establishes confidence and a sense of reliability. If you break it down, there is a pump that pushes fluid through tubes that rest in ground substance. It is not a great mystery.

Some people find it helpful to consider pulse images using physics. For example, total circulating blood volume affects the width of the pulse. This pulse can become turbulent and slippery from pressure on the surrounding vasculature. Possible sources of pressure include masses, tumors, a fetus or a bolus of food.

The ability to identify the standard pulse qualities is essential to best practices. The comparative values of fast-slow, superficial-deep, wide-thin, hard-soft and forceful-weak provide the basic information. Interpretation of this information can be found in all basic Chinese Medical diagnostic texts. However there is a world of impressions that occur in the consciousness based upon the direction in which the attention is placed. It is in the intersection of the observable phenomena and the ephemeral impressions within that we arrive in the possibilities of pulse diagnosis.

23

Five Element Wilderness Walks—Grizzlies and Quicksand

DAVID FORD, LAc *created Taoist Wilderness-Based Five Element Acupuncture to give Acupuncturists additional experiential training in the Five Elements during extensive backpacking field trips through Glacier Bay Alaska, Oregon, and in his native New Zealand.*

Q: How do your "Wilderness Workshops" expand your students' basic knowledge of the Five Elements?

DF: I walk them through each Element, and get them to do different tasks, including tasks they are uncomfortable with—such as being a leader for a day to experience "working with heart" and to overcome shyness, or to do Triple Warmer work (*San Jiao*) in community tasks. We also mix male and female roles, for people with gender role difficulties, for example, men who weren't taught the art of cooking, and women from the cities who never learned wood chopping, get to practice such arts. As much as possible we involve everyone in planning and decision making and legal issues, redefining laws to bend and flex with them (*Wood*—except I don't use that term anymore, I prefer *flora*) or in writing poetry (*Fire)* or in preparing whole foods (*Earth*). The whole emphasis is on getting everyone involved as a family and a team, in a way that allows people to feel safe.

Q: Do you customize your classes to the students or to the environment?

DF: The classes are aimed at professional practitioners but I keep the information basic for lay people, and people who are lawyers, homemakers, MDs and poets. I tell everyone we will be addressing the highest level of learning and that if anybody doesn't understand anything, I'll meet with them in the evening or over a meal. I encourage people with learning or personal challenges to ask me a question 20 times and I'll answer in 20 different ways. These students end up being the best teachers.

Q: How does the concept of "wilderness" strike your city slickers in the group?

DF: They think it's like walking in the park. Then they experience areas in Alaska where the environment is so intense, where the tide changes up to 25 ft, and where there are no cars, no fences, no human influences. We become a part of the landscape. The land walks through us. People living in the cities have a theoretical view of the elements but I think they heal viscerally when they are really in the elements. I try to get people back to the basics, because personally I feel we've lost our roots, we've forgotten that Daoist men and women discovered everything by walking in the environment.

Q: Mention some of the dramatic experiences of the landscape where your students have acquired a new insight?

DF: There was one time in Alaska when we were walking down a trail and noticed exposed tree roots hanging down, and then curling back upwards. David Berkshire said: "look, that's like GB 39" (*Hanging Cup*, also known as *Suspended Bell*). And we all sat down as a class and held that point. Another time, a student got sucked down into quicksand and it took three of us to drag him out. He said he now knew what it was like to experience *Water* overwhelming *Earth* (a feeling of being "stuck").

If you observe rivers and streams, each time the water hits rapids on the way down the mountain, it spins clockwise, then counterclockwise. This is how the Kidneys function in the body. And then there was a time on New Zealand's South Island, in a climate similar to New Mexico, when we were talking about how too much *Fire* and not enough *Water* threatens farming by creating arid climatic conditions.

In Alaska when we observed grizzly bears, I told the group to stand firm, don't show fear (*Water*) don't move, hold their courage, because the bears did not intend to hurt them. As a result, the animals walked away.

Another time, we did a desert meditation on ending nuclear armament, and a rattlesnake climbed into our hands. It was a wonderful example of interspecies communication.

Q: Sometimes you describe the Five Elements as Shamanism!

DF: Five Elements is the Shamanist branch of Asian Medicine. There was a time when a Catholic woman—and a skeptic—came to me during a Wilderness Walk because she was scarlet with hot flashes. I worked Triple Warmer 2 (*San Jiao* 2), and imagined a thunderstorm, and an outrageous hailstorm, and energetically sent freezing cold hail into the point. She felt it instantly!

Q: How do you teach the "Spirit of the Points"?

DF: Some names are very appropriate, like P 6 (*Inner Gate*), and Lu 2 (*Cloud Gate*—that moment in the mountains when the clouds part). But I believe some names are no longer functional. St 36 should be renamed *Great Nourishment* or *Great Garden*. It's very sad for me teaching in TCM schools, where I hear a point referred to as a number, for example Liv 1 (instead of its spirit name *Great Prosperity*). Similarly GB 40 (*Wilderness Mound*) is a metaphor for this point's gift to the body. If you are lost in the wilderness, you find your way by climbing to a high point!

Q: How do you help patients connect with their healing when they don't have the benefit of attending your Wilderness Walks?

DF: I start to educate patients from day one by letting them know that they are in control, I am the student they can fire any time they want to. They should complain about any problems they are having. It's an immediate educational process. I only want to know about their illness as a beginning point. But I also want to know what's beautiful in their lives. Seventy five percent will jump in their chairs; they are so shocked by the question. I am inspired by people's lives and the stories they tell. I also ask patients to tell me when they can feel *Qi,* to be able to get in touch with their own *Qi*. My aim is to get patients out of my office as fast as they can. I have a sign in my office that says: *When you get better—don't blame me!* It's perfect!

Q: *Do your students share stories with you of the ways in which they integrate some of your practical lessons of nature into their healing work with patients?*

DF: They call me back often over a period of a number of years to share life transforming events. Like the practitioner in downtown San Francisco who made a one by six foot indoor garden in her office to grow carrots, lettuce and cauliflower. Or the practitioner in Oregon who takes his patients on nature walks in the park, or the British environmental artist Deborah King who illustrated a children's book based upon her Alaskan wilderness adventure with the bears of Admiralty Island. (1)

Q: *How do you teach Qi?*

DF: The meridians teach me to feel *Qi*. I also teach patients and students to meditate on the points. Sometimes patients describe points vividly. They can feel the energy viscerally. If students have trouble feeling *Qi*, I start with staring exercises, and tell them not to blink. This helps suspend their thinking. I also have them do art, painting, and poetry. I have an ex-army ranger working with me—he's an amazing peace warrior—and he has students walking blindfolded in the woods to heighten their senses.

Q: *What aspects of medicine are modern day students in jeopardy of losing?*

DF: I think we are losing the roots of the medicine. Schools are not nature based anymore. They're based in cities. We should also stop calling ourselves "Complementary Medicine" and use "Traditional Medicine" instead. I'm tired of this "them and us". Our job is to get people better not to get into arguments! Also, schools of Acupuncture are modeling themselves too much on Western Medicine.

Q: *Give us some examples of your best—and worst teachers?*

DF: One of my teachers, J. R. Worsley told me I would learn more from little children and nature, than from any Acupuncture book. My best teachers were curious, had a tremendous sense of humor, had a capacity to move you through emotional states while keeping you personally safe, were full of compassion, and had an open mind and open heart. My worst teachers were those who said there is only one way, and this is the way. They are so enamored with their own belief system they think it's right. I recently saw a great bumper sticker, *Don't believe everything you think!*

Q: Do many people come to your workshops because of compassion fatigue?

DF: I love that term. Yes. Most people come to my wilderness classes because of Compassion Fatigue. I am guilty of it myself. I feel burnt out and them someone calls and says their house is on fire and I think "your house fire is worse than mine" and I treat them. You end up frying yourself in the process.

24

Is that a Cream Pie in Your Face? Songs and Stories in Foundations of Chinese Medicine

BARBRA ESHER LAc, Dipl Ac & ABT (NCCAOM), BFA, AOBTA®-CI
Former President and Director of Education, AOBTA®, and currently a member of the NCCAOM board. Barbra's first degree was in the Fine Arts before she lived and traveled in Asia studying the Asian Healing Arts. She is Curriculum Coordinator and Senior Instructor, Professional Shiatsu and Asian Bodywork Therapy Program, Baltimore School of Massage, Maryland. She practices Acupuncture and Shiatsu in Baltimore.

Q: You are famous for your wonderfully theatrical way of teaching Foundations of Chinese Medicine. Does this reflect your initial training in the Arts?

BE: True, my undergraduate degree was in Fine Arts, and that's inspired a more visual approach and creative thinking—but in Chinese Medicine you need both. Also, many of my students come from artistic backgrounds, they're musicians, writers, visual artists. Chinese Medicine draws on folks with that sensibility. Among my own teachers of Acupuncture there was only one who had any drama or spark and I adored her. She taught Acupuncture theory through stories, and examples from her own life. During the Cultural Revolution she was assigned to be a shoemaker, and soon became a teacher of shoemakers.... so you see, she really had obvious teaching skills.

Q: You inspire your own students to dress up and act out certain pathologies. I've seen one of your students don a Blue Wig, and walk in all wimpy and complaining about lower back pain, and all your other students asked questions and then yelled out "Kidney Yang Deficiency." And a second student came in all blustery with a red angry face and after questioning him and hearing him blast out the answers, they yelled "Liver Yang Rising." You also had a student slap a cream pie in your face while you stood there coughing and spluttering to demonstrate Lung Qi Deficiency at a convention. Can you quote other examples?

BE: Another student walked in with a red face, but his eyes had a wild, distant look, darting here and there, and he said, "sorry, sorry, I just got back from Las Vegas, met a woman in a bar and married her, and haven't slept for a week." Very *Heart Fire Blazing*. And another student brought a sample of dark urine, and another brought a huge container of copious urine, and everyone asked different questions. Everyone knows the Zang-Fu assessments, but no patient fits the definition exactly. In clinic, students come back and say, "oh, this person has a rapid pulse, crazy *Heart Fire Blazing*, let's see if he has a thick yellow tongue coating..... ."

Q: Do you also teach your students Tongue Diagnosis in a theatrical way?

BE: They use food dyes, and that's easy. But they also create tongues out of play dough. Students have taken pieces of fur (yellow—*Heat,* or white—*Cold*) and placed it on their tongues. Others have placed a picture of a yellow coat on their tongue. I let them come up with their own ideas. Some dress up as tongues. Others have brought shells on their tongues to class to reflect scalloped tongues (*Spleen Qi Deficiency*).

Q: How do you teach Pulses?

BE: These are probably the most difficult to illustrate—some draw pulses on the board—others stick pieces of paper on their wrists and show pulses visually. Stephen Birch teaches pulses through a Five Element approach, which I've found to be a most effective way for students to gain confidence. If they find a rapid pulse in the liver position, they immediately hold the Fire Point (Liv 2) on the Liver Meridian and place a red dot on it.

They do this while they are taking the pulse because they can feel the pulse shift immediately—and this validates the connection. If they feel a rolling pulse in the Spleen position, then they take a yellow dot and place it on Sp 3, the *Earth* point which relates to dampness. Similarly, if they feel a slow pulse (cold) in the Kidney position, they put a black dot on K 10, the *Water* point. It's extraordinary how even the beginning student can feel a difference in that pulse. It's a very powerful exercise. Cindy Banker (who developed Five Element Shiatsu) also teaches this approach. It's Japanese, and very effective.

Q: Share some of your other innovations, your use of music, and rhythms?

BE: I love music. I have some sort of song going through my head all day, so it's very natural for me to integrate music into teaching the Five Elements and Eight Principles. For example, while teaching Gall Bladder, and being indecisive, I get them to feel the sides of their body and sing *Should I stay, or should I go?* made famous by *The Clash*. Then the reason why the GB Meridian's on the sides of the body sticks in their heads!

To feel a *Full Heat* condition, I play Peggy Lee's *Fever ("fever in the morning, fever all through the night ... ")* and they remember that *Full Heat* is all day and all night! I play Vivaldi's *Spring* from the Four Seasons, when I teach *Wood*, or Kermit the Frog's *It's not easy being green*. If they can attach their brain to a song, they remember the associations. For *Water*, we sing the blues, or songs about fear, and *Who's afraid of the big bad wolf?*

Then of course for *Metal* there is the Weird Al Yankowitz parody called, *Oops I farted again* (to the tune of the Brittany Spears' *Oops, I did it again ...*) complete with raspberry noises.

Q: What about your use of rhymes and pneumonics?

BE: For Left Pulses, we use the term *HULK* (Heart, Liver, Kidney). For Right Pulses, we use the term *LISP* (Lung, Spleen, Pericardium) For the *Back Shu* (Associated) Points, my student JD came up with: *"Let's Party Hard, Let's Get Some Smoke ... The Kids Love Smoking Bongs ... "* (For Lung, Pericardium, Heart, Liver, Gall Bladder, Spleen, Stomach, Triple Warmer, Kidney, Large Intestine, Small Intestine, Bladder). And for some reason that always sticks in the students' minds....

Q: What other dramatic associations do students use to help them remember?

BE: One student thought about Pirates when she studied *Water*, and all the associations, the ocean, colors black and blue, skull o' crossed bones. In other assignments I use *Winnie the Pooh* characters to express the Elements. Pooh Bear is total *Earth*—very round, yellow, obsessed with sweets ... so I ask my students, "how would you treat him?" Rabbit is a *Woody* control freak, always angry about folks not being on time. Tigger is total *Fire*, enthusiastic, spacy, laughing all the time. We often have arguments about Eyeore and Piglet. Eyeore is gray, and has a mucusy, sadly stuck nature and poor breathing, very *Metal*. Whereas Piglet's primary emotion is fear, and he's small and has very little hair, very *Water*. Then someone suggested salt pork..... .

But I am very much into using figures in the public eye, like the photo of Nick Nolte when he was pulled over for driving under the influence of a drug and appeared totally *Blood Deficient*, dry skin, like a dried up fig. We could almost feel his choppy pulse....

As another assignment I tell students to go into a supermarket, load up their baskets with 100 items, go to the front of the Express line, and then turn around and feel the angry wiry pulse of the folks in line behind them.

Q: What is your favored way of teaching Meridians and Points?

BE: I teach them Yin/Yang first, then the Elements, and only then the Meridians. They must have a vision of how everything fits together. In Asia you always start with the Big Picture and finally whittle down to the details. For example when you mail a letter, you write the country first, then the town, then the street address, and finally the person's name. Much to the annoyance of Westerners, Japanese businessmen will always start a meeting talking about the weather, family issues and only then do they discuss business at the very end. Western businessmen do this the opposite way around. Business first, and then the social stuff.

I've been to Acupressure classes where the first thing they teach is the Points. They go into details before they give a broad picture of where the details fit in. I know an Acupuncture teacher who says if he had to create the whole curriculum all over again, he'd have the students find the Meridians for themselves, to return to the origins of Chinese Medicine. He wouldn't even tell them the locations of the Meridians.... .I think this is a great idea.

Q: If you owned a school of Acupuncture, what changes would you introduce?

BE: More *Touch* from Day One, and an ability to sense Points and develop a Sensitivity around Touch from the beginning. I'd also require a full ABT training to national standards and ideally for ABT board certification, before Acupuncture, and not just a quick weekend introduction. In the USA we're still experiencing a Victorian type of uneasiness around Touch. According to professor Wang who painted our AOBTA® logo, originally there were 12 books in the *Neijing*, two on Acupuncture and 10 on Bodywork. Jeffrey Yuen said that originally the Chinese Bodywork curriculum covered 10 years.

I don't think TCM vilified Touch, I don't blame the Cultural Revolution. I think there is more respect for Tuina in hospitals in China, than here. It's just that the Chinese are imitating Western Medicine by distancing themselves from the patients.

25

New Meridian Discoveries and Directions

TETSURO SAITO, BSc, CST, RMT *is known as the "Father of Shiatsu" in Canada. Originally trained as an electrical engineer in Japan, he had to switch careers on the advice of an eye doctor because of retinal problems, but it was his father who suggested Shiatsu. As a result Tet studied with some of the great 20th century pioneers of Shiatsu development like Toru Namikoshi and Shizuto Masunaga. Later he emigrated to Toronto Canada to create the Shiatsu Center. In recent years his research has focused on new ways of detecting energy and meridian flow. He has documented his Shin So Shiatsu method (translated literally as "deeper level Shiatsu") in two major textbooks books "Shin So Shiatsu" (1) and "Shin So Shiatsu Practitioner's Reference Manual" (2).*

Q: You have pioneered research on meridians and energy flow and discovered new pathways for each meridian. Did your engineering training and knowledge of physics help you develop your sensitivity to energy?

TS: Dealing with the energetic world requires a flexible mind. But my ability to feel *Ki* and meridians developed through Shiatsu and not through my engineering training. A scientific mind can often interfere with the sensibility of *Ki!* However the structuring of my research, my scientific attitude to research and the way I explain my findings to my students does reflect my engineering background. The problem with modern medicine is this—when practitioners cannot see energy, they don't believe in it. But Shin So Shiatsu is a very new approach, just five years old, and some medical doctors are responding to it as it opens up a whole new understanding of how the body works. But I have also discovered the *belt* zones, horizontal zones in the legs we can also use for diagnosis and treatment.

Q: You use Dr Tadashi Irie's "Finger Test" system to feel different qualities of Ki energy and to locate meridians and additional pathways. Why is this, and can you describe it?

TS: Why did I switch to the Irie Method? Palpation of the *Hara* according to Masunaga's diagnostic approach—didn't give me total satisfaction—I didn't have enough confidence in it. So I had to find other approaches to blend with my system of working. I borrowed the "Finger Test" system from a famous Acupuncturist/Pharmacist in Japan—Dr Tadashi Irie—who developed the system as a way of teaching a new diagnostic method to his students, because he felt really frustrated with pulse diagnosis. He wanted to teach a new diagnostic/energetic method that students could see and feel.

Q: Can you describe the Finger Test?

TS: The practitioner places one hand on a meridian or *Hara* zone and diagnoses qualities of energy with the other hand by sliding index finger against thumbnail. The friction produced by this movement is sticky or smooth. The test can be used in many different ways. For example, you could test food through this method. Smoothness means the food agrees with you. Stickiness means the food doesn't agree with you. When you research meridians, stickiness denotes location.

Q: How do you use this method over the Hara?

TS: Let's say you want to check the quality of energy (*Kyo/Deficient* or *Jitsu/Excess*) in the Heart meridian, you point your index finger at the Heart meridian diagnostic zone of the *Hara*, and perform the Finger Test with the other hand, while visualizing qualities of *Kyo* or *Jitsu*. You will feel smoothness if the meridian is *Kyo/Deficient* or stickiness if the meridian is *Jitsu/Excess*. But if the meridian energy is balanced, you will feel neither stickiness nor smoothness, but something in between.

Q: *How do you help your students develop extra diagnostic sensitivity through the Finger Test method?*

TS: The best way to develop sensitivity is to use the finger test every day, on food, vitamins, your own body, your *Hara,* anything. I advise students to practice this method at least ten minutes each day.

Q: *You liken the three different pathways of a single meridian to wires with different capacities for handling electricity. Do you use this imagery and other examples related to electricity to help your students understand your research?*

TS: Sometime yes—they understand the visual comparison.

Q: *Can only Shiatsu graduates with years of experience learn your Shin So Shiatsu method? Or do you feel future students should learn Shin So Shiatsu at the beginning of their training?*

TS: In Canada and in Europe I am only teaching graduates now. But over the last several years I taught the Shin So method from the beginning, and it was often easier for new students to learn the method because they didn't have to break any old patterns or fixed ideas.

Q: *You have said that there are three pathways for each meridian, that the TCM meridian chart abbreviates/oversimplifies the complete meridian system and only shows one of 3 levels of energy, and the third or deepest level of disharmony/imbalance. So what do you say to Acupuncturists and Shiatsu Therapists who have been treating only the most imbalanced meridians and points for centuries?*

TS: That their work will of course help the imbalances in the other pathways, but that they will increase the effectiveness of their treatments by developing a sensitivity to the other pathways. Several Chinese and Japanese Acupuncturists agree that the TCM chart is really an abbreviated, simplified version of a far more complex system and they are developing similar research to explore the additional pathways.

Q: Can you describe a clinical example to show how you use your Shin-So theory to treat a specific patient?

TS: One of my patients came to me with problems in both knees. He'd been to his MD but nothing showed up in his diagnosis. He works in construction and carries heavy loads. And he feels the pain just below the patella area when he walks. I used the Irie Finger Test to locate the source of the problem and there was a sticky sensation over both the lateral and medial sides of both knees. According to the meridian diagnosis there was an imbalance in the extra meridian, and in the deeper system along the Masunaga Spleen meridian—which I would call the third pathway of the Spleen meridian. So in the first session I treated the extra meridian first to balance out the whole energy system. And after that I treated the more local problem using the third pathway of the Spleen meridian. In addition I taped electronic diodes on the most imbalanced structural areas of both knees, to move stagnant *Ki*. As a result his pain dropped after one treatment, when normally this would take two or three treatments. I also noticed a tightness on the inside of his legs, so I showed him a Liver meridian stretch.

Q: You describe the Gall Bladder meridian as an example of a zigzag pattern that, in fact, links each meridian's three pathways.

TS: Yes. The TCM Gall Bladder meridian is the closest reflection of my meridian three-pathway theory.

Q: Are you teaching your Shin So methods to Acupuncturists?

TS: Yes, gradually I'm starting to teach Acupuncturists (Chinese and Japanese). Through the Shin So system they are discovering extra points very easily, and they really appreciate this system. And I am researching points now—by imaging, and they are not related to any meridians. This is the next stage of my research.

Q: You have praised Masunaga's extended meridian system, the basis of his Zen Shiatsu method (3), probably the most popular form of Shiatsu practiced in North America and Europe. But now you say your method goes even further. Both you and Masunaga recognize the flow of meridians throughout the entire body and recognize the TCM chart as an abbreviated version. But now you say all Six Yang Regular meridians begin at Du 20 and at the fingertips, and end at Kidney 1. And all Six Yin Regular meridians begin at Kidney 1 and end at Du 20 as well as at the fingertips. Doesn't this negate thousands of years of Acupuncture theory?

TS: It expands but does not negate the TCM abbreviated chart system! Through the Irie Finger Test I have discovered that all three pathways of each meridian begin and end in the same points, and at the fingertips.

Masunaga's system is somewhere between the TCM chart and my system. He documented the extended system of a flow of the meridians through the entire body, so all the TCM meridians in the legs flow continuously through the torso and arms, and similarly all the meridians in the torso and arms flow continuously through the legs. Zen Shiatsu practitioners usually treat two meridians to correct imbalances in the other ten. Now my system goes even deeper than that.

Q: You have said that, in Japanese culture, enhancing sensitivity in the fingers, and especially fingertips, helps us develop a sharper mind and reduces potential memory loss during the aging process. Japanese Medicine has always placed more importance than Chinese Medicine on touch-as-diagnosis-and-treatment. Does this mean Shiatsu practitioners are less likely to develop Dementia or Alzheimer's?

TS: We hope so! I really believe it helps to use the fingers—it definitely helps—not only on a physical level but it helps the brain as well and this is very important.

26

Roots, Stems and Leaves—Chewing on Chinese Herbs

LESLEY HAMILTON LAc, MSOM, Dipl OM (NCCAOM) *is Academic Adviser and an Instructor of Chinese Herb Studies at the Academy of Oriental Medicine at Austin, where she also co-authored and edited students manuals in Chinese Herbology and Acupuncture Treatment of Disease. She is the creator of Modern World Acupuncture Clinic of Austin. Prior to her training in Asian Medicine, Lesley was a co-owner of a vertical market computer company where she taught small business owners how to use blossoming technology to manage their operations. She also spent years working with horses and their owners, training, teaching and showing. She has sailed in national and international waters and is currently a referee for rowing regattas. From these varied life experiences, she has found many ways to teach difficult subjects, whether she is teaching a rider to bend a horse around the inside leg for a half-pass, or how to trim a sail and set the rudder to hold a direction in a sailboat, or understand the selection of herbs for a particular pathology.*

Q: Many—if not most—western students find Chinese Herbology the most challenging in their training. Chinese Herbology exams often have some of the highest failure rates. Is this because students have problems with rote learning Chinese names? Or do you feel the entire approach to teaching Chinese Herbology needs revamping for a western student?

LH: This is a multi-faceted issue. First one must understand that Asian Medicine is very much like other medical modalities. Memorization of volumes of material is essential. It is neither practical nor efficient for any medical practitioner to look up diseases, diagnoses nor treatments each and every time. The information must be at the forefront of their mind and not buried in deep dark storage!

Memorization of a lot of material requires repetition and then continual use—not unlike learning the vocabulary of another language. I don't believe that for most students learning Chinese pinyin for the herbal substances is any harder or easier than learning common names or Latin names—as most substances are new to the students. Some students come up with their own jingles, jokes, stories and even songs to memorize the lists of names. Some use the Zoo Cards® with pink hippos and purple elephants or make their own colorful flash cards as tools. I like Zhou's study guide *"Chinese Herbology"* (that I co-edited) (1) for the Materia Medica classes because it has been stripped down to the essentials for a beginning student. Bensky's *"Chinese Herbal Medicine—Materia Medica" (2)* and Chens' *"Chinese Medical Herbology and Pharmacology"* (3) are excellent reference books but don't function well for the first layers of memorization. I show students the layers of the memorization process and how to prioritize the layers, and most importantly, to not go onto the next layer until the prior ones are perfected. For example, if they cannot list all the herbs within a category (and its corollary—cannot identify which category an herb belongs to) why learn dosages, cautions and contra-indications or all of the functions?

Then I encourage them to develop a "study-buddy." I suggest they meet for a couple of hours every week and quiz each other. In this way, they use verbal and auditory senses. In addition, they should write short lists, over and over again—using reading and writing skills. This requires different functions in their brain to recall the material in ways they will use on tests, in student clinic and in private practice—speaking, hearing, reading, and writing. Repeat over and over in as many different ways as possible is critical. As old-fashioned as it may seem, memorization is critical to using herbal knowledge. I didn't create rhymes although the occasional funny sounding phrase a classmate came up with worked (herbs to stop bleeding hemorrhoids when said in this order with a questioning and then empathetic tone: *di yu? Huai hua mi?!, Ce bai ye, bai mao gen* ...). I tried using a palm pilot program as a flashcard, but nothing worked better for me than having my study partner say—What are all the release exterior wind-cold herbs? What are the five functions of *huang qin*? I tried the Zoo® cards, but felt like I had to learn someone else's color-picture system and that took too many extra memory bits away from the herbs!

Q: If you were given a free hand to create the Chinese Herbal program for a brand new school—how would you organize this in terms of what you would teach them in the first, second, and third years? AND—how you would adapt the "building block" approach to teaching—single herbs, differentiated, formulas, and patents?

LH: The building blocks of single herbs and formulas and the representative formulas for syndromes leading to their application to disease conditions, makes a lot of sense to me. It is more the teaching methodology within the courses that needs updating for western students. They are often older and have more challenges in their lives (families, jobs, and so on), than their counterparts in China. Because a truly complete herbal studies curriculum takes three years in and of itself, and because it is dependent upon a student's knowledge and understanding of the foundations and diagnostic skills of Asian Medicine, it is necessary to incorporate a sort of continuing education in these basic skills while learning the new herbal material—from year one.

For example, the classifications of herbs do not follow the classifications of the energetics of Acupuncture. The classifications incorporate and cross all the different models—whether Zang-Fu, six stages, four levels, eight principles, six external pathogens, or Five Elements. Unfortunately, students are often still learning the basics of foundations and diagnostics along with the energetics of Acupuncture, when they start to walk down the path of herbal studies.

Q: Which means they sometimes grapple with conflicting information?

LH: Actually, this is not so much conflicting information as it is information that has not fully gelled. Herbal studies often start with herbs that release the exterior—wind-cold and wind-heat. At this point students are only partway through foundations and diagnostics. So I begin by extracting from my students the symptoms that are similar and different in wind-cold and wind-heat—and ask them, what does this presentation look like when the patient comes in the door? Head cold? Allergies? Flu? I have them imagine a picture of this patient in front of them, to visualize the condition, and feel the symptoms from their own personal experiences.

With each new category of herbs, I take a step back and have a dialogue with the students on foundations and diagnostics—in respect to the new category. I often take a historical view of what the herbs may have been used for and then suggest more common current-day presentations. This gives them something to "hang their hat on" before we look at the herb samples. Herbs that are for epidemic febrile diseases—diseases that will not likely walk in their clinic door—have other uses in this day and age. For example, I like to use the four levels when looking at some of the clear heat herbs—in particular the drain fire and cool blood herbs. With four levels, these two categories relate to *Qi* and ying/blood levels. Presentations of severe ying/blood levels that can be seen in epidemic febrile conditions evolving from *wei* and *Qi* levels are not likely to be seen in an American Acupuncture clinic—they should be in the hospital! However, heat in the blood can produce other presentations, such as excessive menstrual bleeding of the perimenopausal women—situations that do walk into the American Acupuncture clinic quite regularly. Again, I combine mild lecture with leading questions to extract these real pictures from the students. The more they develop the picture themselves, the more they will understand and remember.

Q: *What other observations can you share about the way Chinese Herbs are taught today?*

LH: Herbal studies material is very dry. Purely using lecture followed by exams is on its way out in higher education in this country. Some lecture with interactive exercise improves comprehension, retention, and application. A revamping of an herbal studies curriculum would include continual assessment of teaching methodologies to improve the learning outcome. Assessing a student's herbal competency is accomplished formally through written and practical testing, and less formally by the supervisor in the student clinic. As the dialogue between faculty in a school and across schools increases and creative methodologies are shared, I believe we will see increased capabilities of the future practitioners.

I am also a firm believer in developing a tie-in to biomedicine and modern diseases. Most herbal study programs develop an understanding of disease and its treatment in the classics, and Asian foundations. Of course this is extremely necessary, as are the separate studies in biomedicine. However, all too often students and practitioners must make the leap and make correlations between these two distinct medical models by themselves. I do not think this is entirely appropriate. There comes a time in the curriculum where students should be guided around the correlations—the differences and the similarities. I do this to a degree in my classes, being mindful of our legal limitations in the state of Texas.

Q: Can you quote more examples of a biomedical interaction with Chinese Herbs?

LH: A patient with hepatitis C came to me who had been on herbal formulas elsewhere for a couple of years for *Qi* and yin deficiency. This was definitely the Asian Medical presentation. However, his lab tests showed fairly high viral load and stage IV cirrhosis. I tweaked his formula to include draining damp-heat and *Qi* and blood regulating herbs. Several months later his red peeled tongue was nearly normal and he had increased energy. This is one of many examples I use in the class to make the link between the two medicines.

Q: Can you share some other examples with us?

LH: I had another hepatitis C patient with severe ascites. The portal hypertension caused by liver cirrhosis cause the fluid of the blood to be pushed into the abdominal cavity. Diuretics and drain damp herbs no longer had an effect because the water could not get to the kidneys. We opted to try a formula called *Shi Zao Tang* composed of harsh expellants and *da zao*. This forces the water into the intestines causing a watery bowel movement. I warned the patient that it could be extreme! He tried the formula and it worked—he was both relieved and uncomfortable from the experience. That week he was placed on the liver transplant list and had to quit all herbs. I never heard from him again. I have another patient who has mild allergies with mild chronic asthma. He has been on raw herbs for two years—and loves smelling them, looking at them and cooking them—he has incorporated them into his lifestyle. Another was on raw herbs for over a year and doesn't want anything to do with them anymore but likes the customized powders and patents. The key is compliance. Herbs don't help when the patient doesn't take them!

Q: How do you incorporate or apply the wisdom of ancient Chinese Medicine into modern day American lifestyles? How do you make it applicable and meaningful for students preparing to be practitioners?

LH: What a loaded question! This is a book in itself! I approach this on a one-on-one basis with each individual patient. There is no pat answer or one-size fits all mold. I need to know where the patient's perspective is before I can even begin the dialogue—and that is what happens for true healing to begin—a dialogue. As for herbal solutions, often it boils down to patents. I use raw only if the patient is compliant! What is the point if the patient does not have the lifestyle or inclination—or time—to decoct the herbs? Some patients are more open to taking custom formulas of given powders as a choice. However, proof of effectiveness comes with the herbal solution being effective. Patients become repeat customers when the treatment helps them. I incorporate my modern American practitioner adventures and mis-adventures into my classes wherever possible to help students become effective practitioners as well.

Q: What are the other ways in which you bring herbal studies alive?

LH: I *do* agree with other herbal instructors who say that regular testing is important. Students need motivation to review and continue to re-memorize material, and of course exams provide very strong motivation!

Beyond testing, I have a variety of exercises and activities in the classroom that are done in small and large groups. I may have them learn to role model—where one student is the patient with a set of complaints and one is a practitioner who must interview the patient in front of the class. Sometimes the practitioner already knows the herbal answer and then guides the rest of the class to the answer, whereas other times, the class and the practitioner work this out together.

I have scattered the contents of a raw formula in front of students and asked them to identify the components, and figure out what conditions it might be used for (they do not know formulas yet).

Another exercise is to give two to three different groups a disease with three different differentiations. They then establish what the primary symptoms might be for each (for example, diarrhea due to Spleen *Qi* deficiency versus damp-heat versus Kidney Yang deficiency). From that they are to select a half dozen herbs that would be appropriate. Finally they present this to the rest of the class and we discuss the symptoms and the herbs selected. After they do the exercise, I let them know they just learned a strategy for herbal treatment of disease, and that when they are in clinic, they can begin selecting herbs even when they do not yet have formulas under their belt. This both encourages and empowers them to start thinking and not just regurgitating even when they have so much more to memorize!

Q: Given the controversy in China over the marketing of contaminated or fake medications, and foods, and the resulting execution in July 2007 of China's FDA chief, how can you reassure students and patients that your herbal imports are safe?

LH: My herbal products are from reputable companies who follow Good Manufacturing Practices (GMP) Standards. I do not import directly from China. Nor do I purchase from American companies who do not have solid quality assurance practices in place.

Q: What is the best way of planning Chinese Herbal labs?

LH: The first place to start is from budget. What is the purpose of the lab and what is the budget? A wide variety of samples is usually the starting platform—jars, labels, samples, and an adequate supply to refresh the samples from time to time. Identifying, measuring, grinding, keeping some separate from the rest of the formula, and other considerations are commonly covered in an herbal lab. Another possibility would be to pre-prepare in the lab—to "*pao zhi*" (cooking an herb in a special way prior to putting it in a decoction)—and to prepare various substances in the common way—as well as the full decoction of formulations. Dry drying (no additives at all—called "*chao*") is done to *bai zhu* and *bai shao* to enhance their tonifying functions. *Cu zhi* is vinegar frying and is done to herbs such as *xiang fu* and *chai hu* to help with *Qi* regulating and soothing the Liver.

In my labs, we do interactive exercises that may not be "lab" related, but get the students' minds thinking rather than just regurgitating. Again, these may include role-playing patient-practitioner or working in teams to identify the herbs and the function of formula.

Q: Do you believe all students should be required to spend time in the school pharmacy preparing prescriptions for student and professional clinics?

LH: At one time, I did believe this. I certainly believe that the students should have at least all of the Materia Medica classes done prior to working in the school pharmacy. This is as much a safety concern as anything else. In China, students follow a master from start to finish—i.e. they watch and hear the interaction with the patient, see the formulas written and are there for follow-up visits. This provides more complete understanding of herbal application than merely filling formulas in the pharmacy.

Q: *What do students need to have completed in their training to help them understand Chinese Herbal Medicine? Do they need some basic Chinese language training to understand some of the names?*

LH: For identification of herbs, my students learn the pinyin and the Latin words for the parts of plants. Many herb names in pinyin have the part of the plant in the name. If the term for leaf, *ye*, is in the name, they should not identify a root or flower for that name! Also, the pharmaceutical name is an important part of the function. For example, *ma huang* is *herba ephedra* which is the aerial part of the plant, usually the stem. It causes diaphoresis (sweating). But, *ma huang gen* (*gen* means root), *rhizome ephedra*, does the opposite, it stops sweating. I like them to make the connection between the plant name, its function, and the pharmaceutical name.

I also teach them the pinyin names of colors for a variety of reasons. For formulas, they will learn a few words that refer to the action of the formula, but many formulas are a hybrid of the main ingredients' names. If these pinyin words are pointed out, I do not believe very much basic Chinese language is necessary.

Q: *In your labs, do students chew, sniff and sample root, stem and leaves of the different herbs? One student called me in the early hours of the morning with violent diarrhea after a herb class. I told her to talk to the Teacher but also to note the fast moving effects of the herb in future. How do you deal with such reactions?*

LH: My students initially start by tasting the herbs—they always smell and feel them when they look at them. As long as they know the taste of bitter, acrid, sweet, salty, sour and bland, I do not require tasting all herbs. They should take only the very smallest amount to taste. Herbs are typically decocted which would dilute, and sometimes slightly alter, the compounds of the herb. They are not usually ingested raw. Strong or adverse reactions should be expected if ingested raw without preparation—they are not food (not most of them). If I had a student with a strong reaction, I would want to know which herbs were tasted, in what quantity, and what else the student ate in the previous 24–36 hours (as with any medical investigation).

Q: When students come to you for advice prior to training, what would you tell them to expect in Chinese Herbology, and what books would you advise them to read as easy prep?

LH: I tell them to be prepared to memorize and memorize and memorize. I would tell them that Chinese Herbal studies is difficult but do-able, and extremely satisfying for both the practitioner and the patient. I would advise them to review the introductory chapters in Bensky's or Chens' books as a good place to start—after having a solid basis in Asian Medical foundations and medical diagnosis.

Q: The entire Chinese Materia Medica is potentially on the "national test" and I am wondering how you approach studying, or preparing others to study, such an enormous amount of material. Does this differ from the approach needed to be able to practice using the entire Materia Medica?

LH: Consider that the entire Materia Medica is 5000+ substances, and some of us have pared it down to just over 300 herbs! Of those herbs, it could be pared down to the top 175–200 most commonly used herbs. I would focus on those, and allow myself to miss a question on an herb that falls out of those. But *know* those 200 herbs! As for using the rest of the Materia Medica—a practitioner may use those other herbs occasionally—and that is when it is OK to spend some time in research to decide whether to add it in a custom formula for a particular patient.

Q: Of all the Chinese Medical modalities, ingestion of herbs has the greatest potential for causing harm if ingested in toxic amounts, or prescribed incorrectly. How do you convey this responsibility while at the same time encouraging entry level practitioners to utilize the benefits of Chinese Herbal Medicine?

LH: In my first course, each student is assigned an herb to research with emphasis on toxicity, herb-drug interaction, and safety. They must present this information to the class and discuss when to use it and when to avoid it. They learn that the key to safety and efficacy is knowing what else the patient is taking, what the herb's use is, and what the TCM cautions are for the herb. It is a patient-situation by patient-situation call to make.

27

Reflections on Pioneering Chinese Physicians From 5000 BC to 1911 AD

JAN STE.GERMAINE, LAc, MSOM, Dipl Ac, CH & ABT (NCCAOM), AOBTA®-CI *is a former Vice President of AOBTA®, and former Franciscan nun. Jan has taught ABT at Johnson County Community College in the Kansas City metroplex and has mentored Certified Practitioner programs. She practices Acupuncture, Shiatsu and Chinese Herbs in Kansas City. Jan trained in the USA and China.*

Q: Your close-up on the timeline of Chinese Physicians pinpoints information that is not widely known—what inspired you to extract and consolidate the timeline in this way?

JSteG: I was invited by community groups to speak about Traditional Chinese Therapies: Acupuncture, Chinese Herbs, Shiatsu (Asian Bodywork Therapy). Preparing for these, I wanted to cover what kind of treatments they could experience during an appointment in my clinic as well as to motivate them to seek Chinese Medical Therapies for treatment for themselves over other alternative therapies. The yellow pages of every metro area phone book list a plethora of alternative therapies from which to choose. My challenge was to motivate them to choose Traditional Chinese Therapies.

Years ago while doing assigned research at the Midwest College for Oriental Medicine in Chicago, I wrote a paper on Chinese Medical History and Famous Chinese Doctors. I was surprised and impressed by the achievements of early Chinese doctors and amazed at the lengthy timespan of documented Chinese

Medical practice. I decided to include some of that information in my presentation. I considered different ways of organizing the material in a snapshot view and after a few attempts the timeline emerged as a winning format because it placed these famous healers in their historical reality. I could include current events of their day and highlight any relationship they might have had to their dynastic government to make them more real for my audiences.

Among the most impressive Chinese doctors are Zhang Zhong-Jing (142–220 AD) and Hua To (110–207 AD), contemporaries of the second century. Over a ten year period Zhang Zhong-Jing witnessed many relatives die of infectious, contagious, and epidemic fevers. He noticed a definite, repetitive progression of stages of their illnesses and in the midst of his grieving process wrote the medical classic, the *"Shang Han Lun"* (1). His great achievement in this classic is that he identified which Chinese herbal formulas treated which stage of illness. "Zhang was the first to identify the condition of a patient (the diagnosis) with a particular formula used to treat that condition." (2). Some call him the Chinese Hippocrates because he organized signs and symptoms of illness into stages and matched their treatment to certain therapies including herbal formulas such as Cinnamon Twig Soup, Minor Bluegreen Dragon, Buplerum Decoction. I use these herbal formulas in my office with my patients every week. They still work 1,800 years later.

Now HuaTo would approve of the work-out gyms of today being an exponent of systematic exercise which he said expelled bad air. There must have been lots of bad air before the discovery of deodorants and air conditioning. His fame rests on his use of an effervescing powder in wine which acted like anesthesia and was given to patients allowing him to perform many surgeries without causing pain. Unfortunately, the ingredients of this effervescing powder are lost.

Records of his human anatomy studies, surgery and anesthesia were burned upon his death because they transgressed Confucian ideas against "body mutilation". Many ancient civilizations believed cutting a corpse constituted a crime. Writing in the *"World Book Encyclopedia"* (3), Carl C. Francis claims that finally after 400 BC the Greeks allowed rare dissection, and the physician Galen about 100 AD wrote of anatomical structures mostly in animals but also of injured gladiators. The Vatican destroyed many of Leonardo da Vinci's anatomical studies after his death because they transgressed Catholic doctrine of the day. Andreas Vesalius a contemporary of da Vinci who lived decades beyond da Vinci's passing, conducted anatomical studies dissecting bodies of dead criminals and published a book containing a complete description of human anatomical structures when he was a professor at the University of Padua in 1544. He later burned his own writings because he was so maligned by his contemporaries. We truly are blessed to live in an age when the study of human anatomy through dissection is fundamental to medical training.

It is said HuaTo sutured incisions with the thread of medicated mulberry paper and applied a "magic ointment" plaster to the incision that hastened healing. His most famous surgery was on the great general Kuan Yu who had been wounded in the arm by a poisoned arrow. The surgery is celebrated in a painting showing HuaTo incising the injured arm while the general plays chess with his other arm to distract himself from the pain. The information about HuaTo is documented in *"Chen's History of Medical Science"* (4)

Ko Hung, less than 100 yrs later (281–341 AD) lived during the Jin Dynasty, and recorded the world's earliest written description of smallpox and its associated symptoms. Amusingly he doesn't call it smallpox but the "Hun" pox because it was introduced into China when the Huns were fighting the Chinese. It seems the defending Chinese warriors became infected when they came into physical contact with Hun soldiers with the disease.

Remember, the Huns were never able to defeat China, never able to break through the Great Wall and so they went the other direction and ravaged Europe, quite a hike, don't you think? Their great leader Attila threatened Rome but Pope Leo the Great talked him out of it. That was sometime in 452 AD. The encyclopedia says that Attila went home afterwards and died in 453 AD. Maybe the Hun pox?

Sun Szu Mo's (590–682 AD) life spanned both the Sui and Tang dynasties. His understanding of nutrition led him to describe the symptoms of, discover and record the nutritional cure for, beriberi. The first European report on beriberi was in 1642 almost 1,000 years later than the Chinese record left by Sun Szu Mo.

Q: Could you summarize the importance of this information for your students of Chinese Medicine?

JSteG: My commitment to healing through Chinese Medical therapies deepened exponentially as I realized I did not exist in a vacuum but stood on the shoulders of those who came before me. I am just a branch of the giant Chinese Medicine tree. It has deep roots and a long trunk. I found students became grounded and gained confidence in their treatments when, for example, they realized that, for thousands of years, Chinese physicians used the Four Examinations as an interview/assessment method that worked.

Pien Chueh (407–310 BC), one of the earliest Chinese doctors was identified by Ssu-ma Ch'ien in his work *Shih-chi* of 90 BC. Paul Unschuld mentions both Ssu-ma Ch'ien and the *Shih-chi* in his book in the chapter about the origin of the *Nan-Ching (5)* Unschuld says that Ssu-ma Ch'ien wrote a biography of Pien Chueh in *Shih-chi*. Ssu-ma Ch'ien is sometimes called the Chinese Herodotus, because he was the first historian to document Chinese oral traditions of famous medical healers in the *Shih-chi*. Some credit him as the first to organize diagnosis into the system we call the Four Examinations.

Pien Chueh's four diagnostic techniques were: observing, listening and smelling, questioning and palpation. A word about the second examination of listening and smelling. In Chinese, listening and smelling are one word according to Ted J. Kaptchuk (6). But Dr Jamie Wu of the *Academy of Oriental Medicine at Austin*, says, "Ted is partly right. In Chinese, both listening and smelling are called *Wen*. They even have the same pronunciation! Actually, Listening is also usually called *Ting*. This way we use *Ting* for listening and *Wen* for smelling and then there is no confusion." Whether Ting or Wen "smelling" was a much more fragrant olfactory event before deodorant and air conditioning!

Q: How do you use the ancient system of the Four Examinations today?

JSteG: The Four Examinations enable us to look for signs and symptoms of a disharmony. When I observe a new patient, I look at the spirit in their eyes—are they confident, scared, stressed, shy? I also notice their complexion according to their ethnic background of course. Do they have a red face; is it pale, or grey or greenish? Is their expression drawn as when one is in pain, or are they smiling with dancing eyes? Or is their expression blank? What is their body language? I listen to the quality of the patient's voice. Is the volume loud or quiet; is the sound breathy or punctuated by a wheeze? I hear all of this as I listen to the way patients describe their medical complaints.

When I move in their personal space to raise their hand to palpate the pulse or ask them to stick out their tongue, are they comfortable or embarrassed? Their tongues and their pulses tell me about the state of their *Qi* and blood.

These Four Examinations are credited to Pien Cheuh as far back as 90 BC during the time of oral tradition.

Q: When do you share this information with your groups?

JSteG: I introduce the timeline at the first class just to show the roots of TCM. In future when I cover a specific area in TCM class, e.g., meridians, I refer back to the timeline to Wang Wei I (about 1026 AD) and his Bronze Man. Wang Wei I was a court physician in the Song Dynasty (960–1279 AD). He was ordered to compile a handbook on Acupuncture and Moxibustion. Although Acupuncture and Moxibustion had been practiced over a thousand years, information about its structure and practice had been passed from generation to generation by Acupuncturist to apprentice. I'm assuming the dynastic authorities wanted the information documented and concise curricula created to establish national educational standards as well as preserving the information.

In the process of completing his task, Wang Wei I produced a book of drawings of meridian pathways and acupoints. He also cast the famous Bronze Man on which he plotted the meridians and drilled holes on the acupoints. The Bronze Man Model was used to help students learn where to insert the needles. Traditionally, the acupoint holes were filled up with wax and the interior filled with water. I can only imagine that if the student located the points accurately they would be rewarded by getting squirted!

Q: As the chart contains startling information about ancient remedies for, say, smallpox, do you also share the timeline with colleagues in Western Medicine?

JSteG: I had one occasion in which I addressed student nurses who were completing a study of alternative therapies. Yes, I presented the timeline and the students were amazed. They realized Chinese Medicine had been around a long time but hadn't figured it had been around that long.

Q: *The timeline 'personalizes" a lot of otherwise "dry" information. Does this symbolize your approach to teaching Chinese Medicine—to highlight the personalities of individuals throughout the history of Chinese Medicine?*

JSteG: My goal is to connect students with a living Chinese Medicine, to recognize that the methods they are learning or the herbs they are drinking were created and/or formulated by such and such a Chinese doctor maybe a thousand years ago. I want to identify them personally, comment on the historical milieu of their lives and mention any trivia about their lives that would make the students remember them.

Q: *In what other ways has the timeline helped you in your own teaching and in your clinical practice?*

JSteG: In teaching, the timeline provides a matrix, a kind of simple structure, upon which I hang a huge body of knowledge that would otherwise be disconnected and overwhelming. The timeline concept helped me bring these practitioners to life within their historical reality.

In clinical practice, the knowledge of the timeline creates confidence especially when I am presented with complicated cases. Everything I do during a session was contributed by Chinese physicians over 2,000 years ago. They got results so many times using a technique that became part of Traditional Chinese Medical practice. They support and guide me today!

TIMELINE
* FAMOUS CHINESE PHYSICIANS OF THE AGES*

YANGSHAO CULTURAL PERIOD—4000–2500 BC		
Shen Nung—3494 BC	Fu His—2953 BC	Huang Ti—2674 BC

CHINESE DYNASTIES

Shang 1600BC–1066BC	Zhou 1066–221BC	Warring States 403–221BC	Qin 221–206BC	Han Western 203BC–23AD	Han Eastern 25–220AD	Three Kingdoms 220–280AD	Jin 265–420AD	North South Kingdoms 420–581AD
		Pien Chueh			Hua To	Wang Su-Ho	Ko Hung	Tao Hung Ching
					Zhang Zhong-Jing			

Sui 581–618AD	Tang 618–907AD	Five Dynasties 907–960AD	Song 960–1279AD Southern Song 1127–1279AD	Jin Tartar 1115–1234AD	Yuan Mongol 1279–1368AD	Ming 1368–1644AD	Qing 1644–1911AD
Sun Szu Mo			Wang Wei I			Li-Shih Chen	Hsieh Li Heng
			Chang Tzo Ho				
			Li Tung Yuan				

28

What Makes a Great Diagnostician? Quotes from Around the World

Intelligence, humility, and extreme awareness. An ability to listen to everything a patient says. An ability to remember first impressions, and to ask, where is the center of gravity? An ability to keep that center in focus and not allow the mind to be diverted by side effects and symptoms. The greatest practitioners are always ready to go back and look up the basics.
Alan Berman DC, LAc MSOM: Chiropractor and Acupuncturist. Austin, Texas

You have to have a real interest in the **person**, a real interest in "what's there?" You have to trust the richness of the person. One you see this richness you speak differently. You can't fake this. Don't treat patients like "ill people". This isn't theory. It's real. My focus is on what works within the mess—not what doesn't work. If patients see my interest, they feel it's worth it.
Madina Bokoum: Shiatsu Therapist, Counselor and Teacher. Zurich, Switzerland

A good diagnostician collects as much real information about the patient as possible, and that includes not only medical data but also the patient's story of his/her experience of the illness. Thus the diagnostician must interpret both the observable signs of disease and the story of the symptoms. This kind of interpretative skill can only arise through compassionate listening.
Megan Cole MA: Actor of Stage and TV and creator of workshops to teach physician/patient interaction skills to medical and nursing students. Nehalem, Oregon

The ability to work within the framework of a diagnostic system, or more than one diagnostic system, with awareness that the framework is simply a vehicle for tuning into the receiver. Attentiveness and curiosity. Openness and expanded awareness. Respect and honor for the receiver. The ability to interpret one's own experience within a diagnostic system without betraying or modifying that experience.

Carola Beresford-Cooke Lic Ac, MSS: British Acupuncturist and Shiatsu Teacher and author of *Shiatsu Theory and Practice*. Wales, UK

Intuitive sensitivity and a broad deep knowledge base are the two wheels of diagnostic penetration.

Jeffrey Dann PhD LAc, AOBTA®-CI: Acupuncturist, Medical Anthropologist and Teacher. Boulder, Colorado

A superior intellect. A breadth of knowledge. A deep listener. Someone who listens fully and attentively, with some modicum of humility and openness to input from colleagues. Someone who listens to the patient long enough to hear the answers.

Debra Duncan Persinger PhD, DipTchg: Executive Director, Federation of State Massage Therapy Boards. Overland Park, Kansas

Openness in that first contact. The ability to create a supportive atmosphere so the client feels safe. Alignment and presence. The ability to detach his/her own themes from the patient's themes. The ability to reflect, to criticize her/himself, to continue learning, to see and listen to the patient in the widest sense. The ability to see a growth process, and to see the session as an ongoing research process together with the patient in terms of the patient's themes and situation in life. And after a series of sessions, to be able to see the connecting "red line", and for the patient to see those connections in his/her body/mind/spirit.

Anna Christa Endrich: Co-Director, *European Shiatsu Institute*, Heidelberg, Germany

The ability to see people as a great work of art, as a perfect whole. We aren't looking for what is wrong, we want to see more what is right, what is working for them. It is important not to prejudge, and to be really present to seeing people, beyond what they want you to see.

Barbra Esher LAc, Dipl Ac & ABT (NCCAOM), AOBTA®-CI, BFA: Acupuncturist, Shiatsu Teacher, former President and Director of Education, AOBTA®. Baltimore, Maryland

A background in journalism is a superb training for a diagnostician. You learn to read and assess people and situations, quickly and accurately, especially in war reporting. You sharpen intuition when you spend years listening to the unspoken, and observing the invisible. And I always say that physicians and nurses who have worked in the third world make the best diagnosticians, because they have learned to diagnose and treat in the most appalling conditions.

Pamela Ellen Ferguson Dipl ABT (NCCAOM), AOBTA®-CI, GSD, LMT: International Teacher of Shiatsu and Author of eight books. Austin, Texas

A large breadth of theoretical knowledge, highly developed intuition, insatiable curiosity, a healthy desire to be of service, and lots of experience.

Lindy Ferrigno Dipl ABT (NCCAOM) AOBTA®-CI, LMT: Shiatsu Teacher. Charlottesville, Virginia

To be a student, really curious, and a deep listener.

David Ford LAc: Acupuncturist and creator of Taoist Wilderness based training in the Five Elements. Alaska, Oregon and New Zealand

A keen observer. One skilled at observation utilizing as many of his or her senses as possible to the fullest extent possible. Of course the information must be processed in the context of one's knowledge and experience.

Andrew Gamble LAc: Acupuncturist, Chinese Herbologist and Co-Author of *Chinese Herbal Medicine: Materia Medica.* **Massachusetts**

Careful listening. Listening allows me entrée into the deeper realms of the person and therefore the deeper aspect of their nature and the nature of the energetic imbalances and illnesses I will journey with them.

Kathleen Golden LAc, MS: Acupuncturist and pioneer of outreach Acupuncture clinics for disaster zones. New York City

Attention to detail—that's what it comes down to. One of the things I do for pleasure is to read mystery novels—to hone my skills. I'm always looking for the missing piece.

Anne Gray BS, RT(T), LAc, MSOM: Acupuncturist, Feng-Shui Consultant, Austin Texas, and former director, School of Radiation Therapy, Department of Radiation Oncology, Memorial Sloan-Kettering Cancer Center, New York City

A good diagnostician grasps the patient's nature and accurately identifies the root of the imbalance. When I was young, my mother would often take me to business meetings so I could tell her what I thought about everyone there. I just sat back observing facial expressions, body language, speech patterns and tone. It was what I could not perceive with my eyes that gave me the most information. This is the intuitive sense of noticing. At the end of the meeting I would tell my mother my impressions. I was almost 95% accurate.

Karen Greathouse LAc, MSOM, BA (Fine Arts): Acupuncturist and Artist. Austin, Texas, and Mexico City

Pay attention to detail and don't jump to conclusions. For example—hot flashes do not equate Yin deficiency. Don't get wrapped up in the patient's story. Find the questions to ask to arrive at the diagnosis. Know when you don't know. Use biomedical diagnostic techniques when possible and appropriate, but rely on Asian Medicine philosophy and foundations for the diagnoses which provides the treatment plan.

Lesley Hamilton LAc, MSOM: Acupuncturist and Teacher of Chinese Herbology. Austin, Texas

When it comes to making a good assessment, I'd say that, obviously, effective communication skills are a must. You must not only know how to speak with clients, but especially to listen. Listen with your ears, your nose, your mind, your heart, your hands, and your spirit.

Debra Howard Dipl ABT (NCCAOM), AOBTA®-CI, LMT: former President of AOBTA®. New Orleans, Louisiana

A concerned listener. Someone who will take the time for the patient to give the diagnosis from his or her history.

Ed Johnson MD: Professor of Anesthesiology and Pain Management. *University of Texas Southwestern Medical Center,* **Dallas, Texas**

You listen to the story and watch the body language—you take in the whole *gestalt* of patients, how they look, and sound when they answer your questions, not just what they say, but *how* they say it.

Lizbeth Rice Johnson BSN, RNA: Nurse Anesthetist, counselor, and lifetime student of Jung. Dallas, Texas

To know yourself. To be able to deal with your own traumas, fears and taboos. To be neutral and non judgmental. To establish trust. To have professional distance and to know when you are too close to a patient to work with him or her.

To have the ability to admit things you don't know, and to seek information by consulting colleagues, reference books and the internet. To consider diagnosis as a process, and to trust that things reveal themselves when you are open-minded, empathetic, tolerant, patient, and think in new ways. Use of the Five Elements as a diagnostic tool makes you see what you have left out, or ignored.
Beate Johl, Physical Therapist, Shiatsu Teacher and Translator. Berlin, Germany

Being obsessive.
Richard Lewis MD: Nephrologist, Urologist and Transplant Surgeon. *North Austin Medical Center,* **Austin, Texas**

In my mind a good diagnostician continues to learn and practice what he/she has already learned. I do my best intuitive work when I trust what comes up very quickly, a feeling, a thought, an image, a word. I don't think or analyze. Just trust and go with it.
John McKeever: Director, *Shiatsu School Belfast,* **Northern Ireland**

I let the energy of my patient come towards me, she/he will tell me what she/he needs so I will treat accordingly. To be a good "diagnostician" in that way asks me to be relaxed, humble, perceptive in the broadest sense, and welcoming all there is. In short, being exactly the opposite of searching and focusing on something. In this way the flow of energy comes towards me....
Klaus Metzner: Director, *European Shiatsu Institute,* **Munich, Germany**

Having a good grounding in theory and then forgetting theory. Having the ability to see the open door, to see what's in front of you. Often diagnosticians miss the point, they dig too deeply, they make things too complicated, they treat sickness as if it were frustrating, rather than just part of the disharmony pattern.
Lorena Monda LAc, OMD, MS: Acupuncturist, Psychotherapist and Teacher. Albuquerque, New Mexico

Expertise in the basic skills and in the clinical skills of observation, questioning, palpation, listening and olfaction, coupled with a high tolerance for ambiguity, and intuition. Critical thinking is the next piece. A flow chart is an excellent way to work through the seeming contradictions. Intuitions may be recorded in brackets or in a column on the side. Material observations and subjective constructions must be carefully distinguished. This helps to clarify thinking. Diagnosis is enhanced by reflection over time.
William Morris DAOM, MS, LAc: President, *Academy of Oriental Medicine at Austin,* **Texas**

Somebody who is very well trained in their area. Someone who listens with head and heart but also uses his/her eyes. I tell students that the straight A students do not necessarily make the best healers. It's the skilled practitioner who connects with each patient who makes the best diagnostician.
Karen Nunley LAc, MSOM: Acupuncturist and Teacher. Austin, Texas

The ability to listen to patients, respect their individuality, understand not only their health problems but also the impact of the story of their lives.
Thomas Öst LAc, MTOM: Acupuncturist, former board member and Chair of NCCAOM Ethics Committee and Acupuncture Exam Development Committee. Pittsburgh, Pennsylvania

The ability to meet the patient in the moment. To go with her/his *Ki*-movement. To be curious, flexible, and tolerant.
Roberto Preinreich: Director, *European Shiatsu Institute*, Vienna, Austria

In Chinese Medicine we combine many different methods—we need to feel a patient's *Qi*, to observe his/her face and body language. We need to be open minded, use any method available to be able to understand humanity.
Yuxia Qiu MD (China) LAc: Acupuncturist and Calligrapher. Teacher of Acupuncture Techniques, Nutrition, Qigong and Tai Chi. *Academy of Oriental Medicine at Austin*, Texas

The ability to trust and at the same time to be skeptical about yourself and your subjective impressions of the patient. The ability to allow a therapeutic space to unfold freely that is created and shared by practitioner and patient. The ability to show empathy while keeping a therapeutic distance and overview.
Wilfried Rappenecker Dr. Med: Shiatsu Teacher, Physician, and owner, *Shiatsu Schule Hamburg*, Germany

Intellectual clarity, no preconceived opinions. A good knowledge of the five elements and *Hara* diagnosis. A good knowledge of anatomy and Western Medicine, and the ability to bring it all together,
Bernhard Ruhla: Physiotherapist, Shiatsu and Yoga Teacher. Dresden, Germany

Being a Harry Potter groupie! Every time the publication of a new book or movie in the series is imminent, I re-read all the former books in order. I make a note of scenes and facts I forgot after reading that work for the first time, as a way of reminding myself to be alert to the signs and symptoms I may have forgotten or overlooked in a new patient. This is how I rationalize the hours I spend reading the books. They train me to be alert. My garden also trains me to be alert and aware of growth patterns and setbacks and how to diagnose and nurse ailing vegetables and herbs to help them thrive!

Jan Ste Germaine LAc, AOBTA®-CI: Acupuncturist and Shiatsu Teacher. Former vice president AOBTA®. Kansas City, Missouri

There are no short cuts. Masunaga *Sensei* taught us to shut out the brain when diagnosing. To become good diagnosticians we need to develop *Hara* and *tanden*—the second brain, dealing with the energetic system. We need to develop high *KI* energy through daily practice—following the basics—mind, posture, breath—these 3 aspects, together with meditation, Tai Chi or Qigong. But to be a good diagnostician also requires years of experience.

Tetsuro Saito BSc, RMT, CST: known as the "Father of Shiatsu" in Toronto, Canada

A lot of knowledge, humility, curiosity, open mindedness, boldness, being tuned to the evidence that is "not present" (the untold or unseen), mindfulness and meditative faculties.

Elad Schiff MD: Chair, Unit for CAM, Integrative Medicine, Law & Ethics, Haifa, Israel

Someone who possesses a great deal of knowledge and is continually learning more. Someone with excellent communication skills, particularly in the areas of listening, reflective feedback, and eliciting accurate information. A good diagnostician weaves her assessment with the client's verbal information to determine the true condition.

Cherie Sohnen-Moe BA: Teacher, Healing Arts Practitioner and Co-Author *The Ethics of Touch,* **Tucson, Arizona**

The most important thing is openness toward a patient, and a big heart, because this is how you perceive more. At the same time you also need detachment because too much heart and empathy can cloud the picture. A lot of life experience and a lot of clinical experience also helps diagnostic perception.

Edith Storch: Shiatsu Teacher and owner, *Shiatsu Zentrum Edith Storch,* **Berlin, Germany**

A good diagnostician is one who develops an ability to see the intricate patterns and transitions of Yin and Yang in an individual and in the environment. And understands the interplay of the two. By seeing the momentum of the pattern and its ever changing dynamic, the good diagnostician can begin to understand the force needed to slow the progression or stop the decline of a patient's health, thereby becoming a good healer or harmonizer.

Maryanne Travaglione LAc: Acupuncturist and Teacher, Brooklyn, New York

To be a good diagnostician is to have two points of view at the same time. One eye (left hemisphere) notices all the details, and the other eye (right hemisphere) gets an impression of the whole. Then it is necessary to bring those two sights together—to complete the whole impression with the details, and to evaluate the details according to the whole impression.

Eduard Tripp DPhil: Psychotherapist, Shiatsu Teacher, Editor, Vienna, Austria

The most important quality for a good diagnostician is humbleness—the ability to refrain from making quick and rigid judgments and to keep an open mind. You need to keep your eyes and ears open for new information from the client's body, words or actions. Don't assume that you know what the problem is or how to fix it. Ask questions and listen carefully to the answers. Diagnosis starts at the first contact with the client and continues through to the end of the treatment and the final 'good-bye'.

Nancy van der Poorten, BSc, CST: Vice-Principal Emerita, *Shiatsu School of Canada*, and currently studying butterfly ecology in Sri Lanka

One who gets the diagnosis right most of the time. There are so many ways to diagnose a problem. Personally I think the practitioner who uses a lot of touch comes to good conclusions. A good diagnostician also communicates well.

Stuart Watts LAc, AOBTA®-CI: creator of schools of Asian Medicine. Austin, Texas and Sante Fe, New Mexico

A combination if wisdom and good training in many different disciplines and an openness to new discoveries. A good diagnostician also learns a lot from their patients, and from exchanges with colleagues. I benefit from my medical studies, my studies in complementary medicine and my singing.

Carien Wijnen Dr. Med: Dutch born Physician, choir teacher. Berlin, Germany

Experience, Compassion, listening with all your senses, eyes, ears, nose and touch. But when you're dealing with a patient who is a constant complainer, it's dangerous to think, "it's the same old story." You must look at the patient with a new eye each time.
Bernadette Winiker RN, CCTC: Transplant Supervisor. *North Austin Medical Center,* **Austin, Texas**

"Practice, practice, practice"! Only when we practice in clinic, can we skillfully apply diagnostic techniques and methods. We should know 28 types of pulses, and all their characteristics and indications.
Qianzhi (Jamie) Wu MD (China), LAc, AOBTA®-CI: Faculty Dean and Director, Integral Studies. *Academy of Oriental Medicine at Austin,* **Texas**

A good diagnosis is based on experience, that's why practitioners of Chinese Medicine need a lot of practice. The more cases they see, the more experienced they become. A good foundation of didactic and clinical training is vital. Otherwise, there's no substance. **Zheng Zeng MD (China), LAc: Teacher, and Director of Acupuncture.** *Academy of Oriental Medicine at Austin,* **Texas**

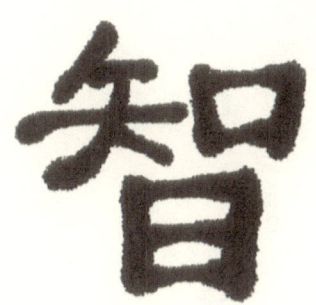

WISDOM—calligraphy by Yuxia Qiu, LAc

References

TEACHERS HERE, THERE AND EVERYWHERE

www.brainyquote.com quotes from Anais Nin (1) and Leonardo da Vinci (2)

CHAPTER 5

1. Ferguson, Pamela (1995): *The Self-Shiatsu Handbook,* Berkley-Perigee, New York City.

2. Ferguson, Pamela (2000): *TAKE FIVE—The Five Elements Guide to Health and Harmony,* New Leaf/Gill & Macmillan, Dublin, Ireland.

3. National Public Radio (Morning Edition): *Former Soldier Helps Others Fight Army for Help:* July 7 2007. *Pentagon Report Cites Mental Health Care Concerns:* July 7 2007: *Gaps in Mental Care Persist for Fort Carson Soldiers* May 24 2007, *Military Mental Health Care Under Scrutiny:* March 6 2007.

CHAPTER 7

1. Salvo, Susan G. (2006): *Massage Therapy Principles and Practice (second edition)* Elsevier, New York City.

2. Braun, Mary Beth, and Simonson, Stephanie J (2007): *Introduction to Massage Therapy (second edition),* Lippencott Williams & Wilkins, Philadelphia, PA.

THE WORKPLACE

1. McCourt, Frank (2005): *Teacher Man:* Scribner, New York City.

2. Sacks, Oliver (1995): *An Anthropologist on Mars: Seven Paradoxical Tales,* Alfred A. Knopf, New York City.

CHAPTER 11

1. Rappenecker, Wilfried (1997) *Yu Sen:* Felicitas Hubner-Verlag, Germany.

2.   Rappenecker, Wilfried (1998) *Funf Elemente und 12 Meridiane:* Felicitas Hubner-Verlag, Germany.

3.   Rappenecker, Wilfried, and Kockrick, Meike (2007) *Atlas Shiatsu—Die Meridiane des Zen Shiatsu:* Urban-Fischer (Elsevier) Verlag, Germany.

LOOKING EAST—FACING WEST

1.   Walker, Brian (1992) : *Hua Hu Ching—The Teachings of Lao Tzu:* Clark City Press, Livingstone, MT.

2.   Mitchell, Stephen (2006): *Tao Te Ching—Lao Tzu (latest translation) :* Harper Perennial Classics, New York City.

CHAPTER 16

1.   Mehrabian, Albert (1972): *Non-Verbal Communication:* Aldine-Atherton, Chicago Illinois.

2.   Savitt, Todd L. (2002): *Medical Readers' Theater: A Guide and Scripts:* University of Iowa Press, Iowa City, Iowa.

CHAPTER 17

1.   Monda, Lorena (2000): *The Practice of Wholeness: Spiritual Transformation in Everyday Life:* Golden Flower Publications, Placitas NM.

2.   Monda, Lorena, with Scott, John (2005): *Clinical Guide to Commonly Used Chinese Herbal Formulas:* Herbal Medicine Press, Placitas NM

CHAPTER 18

1.   Sohnen-Moe, Cherie (2008): *Business Mastery (4th edition):* Sohnen-Moe Associates, Inc. Tucson, AZ.

2.   Sohnen-Moe, Cherie, and Benjamin, Ben PhD (2003): *Ethics of Touch:* Sohnen-Moe Associates, Inc. Tucson AZ.

ECLECTIC METHODOLOGY

1.   Humphreys, Christmas (1996): *Zen Buddhism:* Diamond Books, London UK.

2.   Phillips, Christopher (2001): *Socrates Café:* W.W. Norton & Co, New York City.

CHAPTER 22

1. Scheid, V. (2007). *Currents of Tradition in Chinese Medicine 1626–2006*. Eastland Press, Seattle WA.

2. Wang, B. (1997a) *Yellow Emperor's Canon of Internal Medicine*: China Science and Technology Press, Beijing, China.

3. Wang, S. (1997b). *The Pulse Classic a Translation of the Mai Jing*: Blue Poppy Press, Boulder, CO.

4. Wei, J. (1997). *The Practical Jin's Pulse Diagnosis*. (L. Yubin, Z. Rong & M. Xinyuan, Trans.). Shandong Science and Technology Publications: Shangdong, China.

5. Maciocia, G. (1997) *The Foundations of Chinese Medicine: A comprehensive text for acupuncturists and* herbalists: Churchill Livingstone. Great Britain.

6. Zhen, L. S. (1981). *Pulse Diagnosis*. (H. K. Huynh, Trans.): Paradigm Press. Brookline, MA.

7. Kaptchuk, T. (2000). *The Web That Has No Weaver: Understanding Chinese Medicine:* Contemporary Publishing Group, Chicago, IL.

8. Cheng, X., & Deng, L. (Eds.). (2005). *Chinese Acupuncture and Moxibustion.*: Foreign Languages Press, Beijing, China.

9. Deng, T. D. (1999). *Practical Diagnosis in Traditional Chinese Medicine:* Churchill Livingstone. Great Britain.

CHAPTER 23

1. King, Deborah (2002): *Bear's Dreams Picture Book,* Harper Collins Ltd, London UK.

CHAPTER 25

1. Saito, Tetsuro (2006) : *Shin So Shiatsu,* Trafford Publishing, Victoria BC, Canada.

2. Saito, Tetsuro (2006) : *Shin So Shiatsu Practitioner's Reference Manual,* Trafford Publishing, Victoria BC, Canada.

3. Masunaga, Shizuto, with Ohashi, Wataru (1977): *Zen Shiatsu, How to Harmonize Yin and Yang for Better Health,* Japan Publications. Distributed by Harper & Row, New York City.

CHAPTER 26

1. Zhou, Z (2003) *Chinese Herbology: A Student Study Guide (2nd edition)* Austin AOMA Press.

2. Bensky, D., Clavey, S., Stoger, E., Gamble, A., and Bensky, L. L. (2004) *Chinese Herbal Medicine—Materia Medica (3rd edition)*: Eastland Press, Inc., Seattle, WA.

3. Chen, J. and Chen, T. *Chinese Medical Herbology and Pharmacology.* (2004). Art of Medicine Press, Inc., City of Industry, CA.

4. Sionneau, P. (Translated by Flaws, Bob.) (1995) *Pao Zhi—An Introduction to the Use of Processed Chinese Medicinals,* Blue Poppy Press, Boulder, CO.

CHAPTER 27

1. Zhang Zhong-Jing, (1981) *Shang Han Lun: Wellspring of Chinese Medicine,* edited by Hong-Yen Hsu, Ph.D and Willian G Peacher, M.D, Keats Publishing, Inc and Oriental Healing Arts Institute, Long Beach, CA.

2. Bensky & Barolet, *Formulas & Strategies,* (1990) Eastland Press, Inc., Seattle, WA.

3. Francis, Carl C. (1972) *Anatomy Article—World Book Encyclopedia,* 1972 Field Enterprises Educational Corporation, Chicago IL.

4. Drs. *Hong*-Yen Hsu and W. Peacher (1977) *Chen's History of Chinese Medical Science,* Oriental Healing Arts Institute, Long Beach, CA.

5. Paul U. Unschuld, translator, (1986) *Nan-Ching The Classic of Difficult Issues,* University of California Press, Berkeley and Los Angeles, CA.

6. Kaptchuk, Ted. (1983) *The Web That Has No Weaver,* Congdon & Weed, Inc, Chicago, IL.

Additional Reading List

We'd like to share a selection of the works we discussed or discovered during the evolution of *Sand to Sky*. These were written by teachers and by physicians who "think outside of the box" and crafted unusually inspiring stories around their respective insights, and experiences. Books with an asterisk* were made into movies.

By Teachers: Even though most of the following works deal with school—and not college level teachers—some of the inspired methodology, breakthroughs and insights transcend all ages. It's often useful for teachers of adults to gain insights into behavioral patterns that may be rooted in middle or high school experiences. Similarly it is always inspiring to read about teachers who have turned students' lives around through persistence and spontaneity. You won't find the following collection of stories and anecdotes in textbooks on education!

*Albom, Mitch. (1977) *Tuesdays with Morrie: An Old Man, a Young Man, and Life's Greatest Lesson.* Doubleday, New York.

*Conroy, Pat. (2001) *The Water is Wide.* The Dial Press, Random House, New York, 2002 or via e-books from RosettaBooks, New York City.

Esquith, Rafe: (2007) *Teach Like Your Hair's on Fire: The Methods and Madness inside Room 56.* Viking Penguin, New York City.

Jones, Lloyd: (2007) *Mister Pip.* The Dial Press, New York City.

Karg, Barb, and Sutherland, Rick (2006) *Letters to My Teacher.* Adams Media Corporation, Avon, MA.

Mortenson, Greg and Relin, David Oliver (2007): *Three Cups of Tea—One Man's Mission to Promote Peace One School at a Time.* Penguin Books, New York City.

McCourt, Frank (2005) *Teacher Man*—Scribner New York City.

*The Freedom Writers with Gruwell, Erin (1999): *The Freedom Writers Diary—How a Teacher and 150 Teens Used Writing to Change Themselves and the World Around Them.* Broadway Books/Doubleday, New York City.

*Warren, Larkin, and Guaspari, Roberta (1999): *Music of the Heart—the Roberta Guaspari Story.* Miramax Books, New York City.

And additional movies:

- Bennett, Alan: *The History Boys* (the movie is based on the award winning play)
- *Mad Hot Ballroom*
- *Dead Poets Society*
- Holland, Glenn. *Mr Holland's Opus*

By Physicians: *Similarly, we wanted to share works by physicians offering poetic, insightful and unusual insights on everything from a cadaver lab, to the inner workings of a practitioner's mind, to maverick ways of diagnosing and treating patients. Whether your focus is on Asian or Western Medicine or a creative integration of both, you'll find these stories inspiring.*

Chen, Pauline (2007): *The Final Examination: A Surgeon's Reflections on Mortality.* Alfred A. Knopf, New York City.

Firlik, Katrina (2007): *Another Day in the Frontal Lobe—a brain surgeon exposes life on the inside.* Random House Trade Paperback, New York City.

Gawande, Atul (2007): *Complications—A Surgeon's Notes on an Imperfect Science.* Picador New York City.

Groopman, Jerome MD (2007): *How Doctors Think.* Houghton Mifflin, New York City.

Montross, Christine (2007): *Body of Work—Meditations on Mortality from the Human Anatomy Lab.* The Penguin Press New York City.

Roach, Mary (2004): *Stiff: The Curious Lives of Human Cadavers.* Norton Paperback New York City.

*Rosenbaum, Edward E (1988). *A Taste of My Own Medicine—When the Doctor is the Patient* (filmed under the title "The Doctor") Random House, New York, 1988.

Sacks, Oliver:
The Man Who Mistook his Wife for a Hat: and other clinical tales (1998). Touchstone, New York City.
An Anthropologist on Mars: Seven Paradoxical Tales (1995). Alfred A. Knopf, New York City.
Island of the Colorblind (1996) Alfred A. Knopf, New York City.
Migraine (1992) Vintage Books, New York City.
Awakenings (1990) Harper Perennial, New York City.
A Leg to Stand On (1998) Touchstone, New York City.
Seeing Voices. (2000) Vintage Books, New York City.
Uncle Tungsten (2000) *Memories of a Chemical Boyhood.* Vintage Books, New York City.
Musicophilia (2007) *Tales of Music and the Brain.* Alfred A. Knopf, New York City.

Glossary

USA

AAAOM: *American Association of Acupuncture and Oriental Medicine*
www.aaaom.org

ACAOM: *Accreditation Commission for Acupuncture and Oriental Medicine*
www.acaom.org

AOBTA: *American Organization for Bodywork Therapies of Asia*
AOBTA®-CI—Certified Instructor www.aobta.org

CCAOM: *Council of Colleges of Acupuncture and Oriental Medicine*
www.ccaom.org

FSMTB: *Federation of State Massage Therapy Boards*
www.fsmtb.org

NCCAOM: *National Certification Commission for Acupuncture and Oriental Medicine*
Dipl. ABT (NCCAOM): Diplomate in Asian Bodywork Therapy
Dipl. Ac (NCCAOM): Diplomate in Acupuncture
Dipl. CH (NCCAOM): Diplomate in Chinese Herbology
Dipl. OM (NCCAOM): Diplomate in Oriental Medicine. www.nccaom.org

NOCA: National Organization for Competency Assurance, and its accreditation body, NCCA: National Commission for Certifying Agencies www.noca.org/ncca/ncca.html

NQA: National Qigong Association www.nqa.org

CANADA

STAO: *Shiatsu Therapy Association of Ontario*
www.shiatsuassociation.com

EUROPE

GSD: *Gesellschaft für Shiatsu Deutschland (German Shiatsu Society)*
www.shiatsu-gsd.de

SGS: *Shiatsu Gesellschaft Schweiz (Swiss Shiatsu Society)*
www.shiatsu-sgs.ch

ODS: *Österreichischer Dachverband für Shiatsu (Austrian Shiatsu Society)*
www.shiatsu-verband.at

The Shiatsu Society (UK)
www.shiatsusociety.org

Schools:

USA

AOMA: *Academy of Oriental Medicine at Austin:* www.aoma.edu
ASAOM: *Arizona School of Acupuncture and Oriental Medicine:* www.asaom.edu
Baltimore School of Massage: www.steinered.com
DIHA: *Desert Institute of the Healing Arts:* www.diha.edu
PCOM: *Pacific College of Oriental Medicine:* www.pcom.edu
SWAC: *Southwest Acupuncture College* www.acupuncturecollege.edu
TOURO: *Touro College:* www.touro.edu
TSCA: *Tri-State College of Acupuncture:* www.tsca.college-info.com

Programs—*Awakening to the Soul of our Medicine*: www.asomseminars.com

EUROPE

Germany

Shiatsu-Zentrum Edith Storch: www.shiatsu-zentrum.de
*Europäisches Shiatsu Institut—ESI Munchen—*www.shiatsu.de
*Europäisches Shiatsu Institut—ESI Heidelberg—*www.shiatsu.de
*Schule für Shiatsu Hamburg—*www.schule-fuer-shiatsu.de

Switzerland

Flying Ki Shiatsu School: www.lorengo.ch
Kientalerhof: www.kientalerhof.ch

Austria

Europäisches Shiatsu Institut—ESI Austria: www.shiatsu-institut.at

Afterword

Sand to Sky will no doubt prompt more questions than it answers. We hope the conversations will inspire dynamic classrooms and more Teacher training. We also encourage the respective associations to offer workshops and panel discussions by and for Teachers at future conventions.

We would love *Sand to Sky* to stimulate ongoing exchanges between Teachers of Asian Medicine across the world. May the conversations continue.

Yours in *Qi*

Debra and Pam
sand2sky@gmail.com

978-0-595-44515-8
0-595-44515-2

www.ingramcontent.com/pod-product-compliance
Lightning Source LLC
Chambersburg PA
CBHW030309290526
45785CB00001B/276